With Steadied Hands

Selected and new medical poems

by John Manesis

With Steadied Hands

"The best doctors in the world are Doctor Diet, Doctor Quiet, and Doctor Merryman."

Jonathan Swift

Acknowledgments

Among the journals which have included my poetry of are the following publications:

Zone 3, Mediphors, Forkroads, Poetic License, Black Creek Review, Footwork: Paterson Literary Review, Dream International Quarterly, North Coast Review, Wisconsin Review, Poetry Motel, Second Glance, Creighton Window, Nebo, California State Poetry Quarterly, Bay Area Poetry Coalition, Loonfeather, Opus Literary Review, Minerva, Lake Region Review, Mayo Magazine, Touched by Adoption(by Green River Press), The Cancer Poetry Project(by Fairview Press), Winterhawk Press, Pella Publishing, Whispering Angel Books, University of Evansville Press, Baseball Bard, and Extra Innings.

My thanks to the editors.

Contents

Other Candle Lights (2008)

Consider, If You Will (2010)

In the Third Season (2012)

New Poems

For Bess

For Mary, Stephanie, George and Peter

With All My Breath (2003)

A Beginning

The anatomy professor
ushered our student retinue
into the large dissection room
as light slanted through the windows
that autumn afternoon.

Bespectacled and reverent,
he called our names and assigned
a foursome to each cadaver
where we, the acolytes, would serve
the coming year at medicine's altar.

After initial anxious moments,
we lifted up our instruments
that gleamed in halos of suspended lamps
to study muscles, nerves, vessels and bones--
the covers and bindings of their books.

Since then I've come to ask myself
about the missing words and sentences,
the blank pages of their days.
Where did their travels take them,
did anyone record their stories?
How many went unclaimed,
who among them willed away the last,
perhaps the only thing they owned?

The Right Time

Thirty years ago my cousin,
shackled by delusions and despair,
was taken to an asylum
on the island of Corfu,
not far from his birthplace.

A doctor asked him,
"What is your name?
Where were you born?
What day is it?"
When there was no answer,
the doctor scribbled a few lines
on a blank sheet of paper
and closed the chart.

Days passed into years, one brick
laid upon another, row on row,
and by the time four walls rose
above his head my cousin,
numbed by tranquilizers, had quit
bloodying his fists against the stone.

But every night, before he dropped
into a well of fitful sleep he pressed
an ear to the wall and listened

to the outside world he remembered--
the plaintive strings of a bouzouki,
his mother humming in the kitchen,
wine glasses clinking in a cafenio.

After spending half his life confined,
he collapsed and in that final hour
as he was borne away looked upward,
saw a small square of blue sky and said,
"I know what day it is."

Arseni Manesis

You see the way I am?
My strength is gone
and I can't walk no more--
the doctor calls my sickness MS.

I remember how it started--
1936 at your father's wedding.
No feeling in my right hand
and no matter how hard I try
I can't tie my own shoes so I ask
your aunt who does it for me.
She thought I made a joke.

Five years before I got sick
my friend, Nick, from same village
in Greece, came to Chicago and found
pretty young woman he wants to marry
but he already has wife and two boys
in old country waiting for him to come back.
He says to me, "Arseni, you stand up for me—
I need witness to say I am good man,
not married, that you know me from Greece.
Don't worry, they will believe you--
I make it up to you later on."

In front of God, I raised my right hand
but inside I knew it was wrong, a lie.
Funny thing, they were never happy,
never good for each other
and after two years she leaves him.
You see now how this happened,
why the sickness start in my right hand?
My own fault, nobody else.
God knows.

In a Room Upstairs
-for Yiayia

When my grandmother struck a match
and lit a candle next to the icon,
the coat hanging in the corner
no longer resembled an intruder.

She sat beside me on the bed,
and murmured a prayer in Greek,
only part of which I understood,

crossed herself and made the same sign
on my forehead and hands,
her fingertips warm and steady.

Not having to say anything else,
she returned to the kitchen
and I fell asleep listening to
the sound of her slippered feet.

I don't remember what ailed me--
some fifty years have passed--
and yet whenever I summon her,

she ascends the stairs,
the candle still glows,
soft and low, and her light
brightens my darkest nights.

Reflection

Naked,
the teenager stands
sideways before a mirror,
ignoring her mother's pleas
at the bedroom door.

She cranes to inspect
the shriveled breasts and studies
her ribs, flared as a swan's back.
With one hand on her spine,
the other against her abdomen,
she measures herself.

When she turns to face
the reflection in the glass,
she remembers the carnival,
the low and narrow corridor
and other girls laughing
at contorted faces and wide torsos.

She hears the last meal—
a bite of an apple—
churning above the navel
like water on the rise.

Graven Images

"I no longer wanted to be an artist."
Beto de la Rocha, *L.A. Times*

The painter slashed every canvas,
smashed the wooden frames
and torched his life's work
as though his soul was afire.
"But why?" his friends asked--
"Because I loved my art
more than God," he explained
and withdrew from the world.

For twenty years he searched
the Scriptures for an answer,
memorizing verse after verse.
When he lay upon the cot
and closed his weary eyes,
mad Nebuchadnezzar appeared,
babbling in the fields,
clouds of locusts swirled into Egypt,
Job's sores and blisters wept.

One night, deep in a chasm,
pressed against the dank walls,
over and over he yelled
for someone to raise him up
but the only sounds he heard

were the echoes of his own voice.
He understood what he had to do
and began the steep ascent,
inching upward, his swathed hands
clawing at the earth's mossy bones--
the dirt, stones, rocks, bare roots.

He awoke then,
drew back the shades
and waited at the window.
Morning finally came,
a garden of hues on the horizon
blazing with lilacs, roses, and blues
and as he watched the sun rise
relived the light in his landscapes.
The painter took up his brush again.

Rehearsal

With the lights low,
she glances at the mirror
as though it were an audience,

tells herself,
I know my lines by heart--
a little more makeup now

and I can go to the store.
When he comes home,
he'll hand me a bouquet,

a card with the right poem,
and we'll be passionate tonight.
He shouldn't have done it--

if someone asks why this happened,
I will remember what to say,
the part that I'm supposed to play.

I'll give him one more chance--
deep down I know he loves me
the way he always has.

Freed

Fear, a constant companion,
dogged the boy to school,
snapping at his pant legs--
called upon in class to speak
the more he fractured words,
the more protracted the pauses,
the more consonants clung to his larynx,
baffles in turbulent streams of air--

and so his voice inverted,
deeper than the swirls and coils
of his inner ear but when he dreamed
he saw himself seated in a great hall,
the teacher aiming a finger at him--
as the schoolboy rose,
classmates leaned forward, hushed--
he uncupped his hands and freed
a swallow that swept around the room
until it found a window
open to the world of sound.

Gone

On a deserted platform
beside the railroad station,
the old man stares up
at the still black hands
of the clock that faces west
high atop the depot tower.

Unforgettable

After killing a trainer and escaping from a
circus, an elephant named Tyk was shot on a busy
street.
                    Honolulu, AP Press, August 21, 1994

"Why did she go berserk?"
the veterinarian mused,
probing several of the bullet holes
as he circled the carcass,
studying it from trunk to tail.

He excised the eyes,
gazed at them under a microscope
and saw not the savanna's wide sky
but flashes from a thousand cameras
imprinted on the retinae.

He lifted the huge pinnae,
listened at the ear holes
and heard not the song of the wind
along the Serengeti but the sounds
of cymbals crashing and balloons
popping like a rifle regiment.

He cut away the ribs,
descended into the depths
of the thoracic cage and there

discovered the last birthday cake,
shaped like an elephant's heart,
the icing topped with peanut butter
and twenty-one carrot sticks.

Wen

The first time we made rounds
as junior medical students
at the Omaha V.A. Hospital,
we crowded behind Dr. Kleitch,
a handful of foot soldiers
in the company of a General.
The conversations on the ward
came to a halt in mid-sentence
as he made his entrance,
a compact surgeon with grey hair
that bristled, wire rimmed glasses
and eyes glinting like ball bearings.
He stopped to examine a patient
who dangled his feet over the bed.
Dr. Kleitch pointed to a lump
on the man's forehead and asked me,
"What's that, Doctor?"
I stared at the swelling,
hoping in vain it would somehow
reveal its mysteries to me,
and replied, "I don't know."
"You don't know? I am sure even
he knows," the surgeon proclaimed,
glaring at the patient who gulped,
cleared his throat and said,
"Sorry, me neither, Doc."
I thought I saw a faint smile

trying to escape from the corner
of our leader's mouth.
"It's a wen...spelled, W..E..N,
a sebaceous cyst, Doctors,
benign, well circumscribed,
non-tender, soft, and commonly seen
on the face, scalp or back.
Don't ever forget it!"
I survived that initiation,
my boot camp, with a flesh wound
but no internal injuries.
To this day, whenever I see a wen,
the curtains of the past part,
Dr. Kleitch strides onto the stage
and there I am in the front row,
lucky to have a ticket to the show.

Tremor

The young adult, hunched in a chair,
fists on his knees, queried me,
"Why does every pipe I grab
at work turn to rust the next day?
When I asked Doc Lemay,
he laughed at me," the man said,
his eyes like grey stones
at the bottom of a cold creek.
Selecting words the way
an expert in explosives
handles a suspicious package,
I explained the composition of sweat,
delayed effects of humidity,
the way that metals oxidize--
a solemn oration of gibberish.
An eerie calm came over him
and his hands fell to his side.
Nodding, he left the office
and I never saw him again.
Now, twenty five years later,
I wonder if he felt the rumble,
the fault lines shifting in his life,
if I should have helped him see
the cracks angling beneath his feet
instead of running for safer ground.

Whatever Happened to Zack,

the only black man in town?
Coal colored face thrust forward,
his head gleaming like an eight ball,
he would stop us on the street,
pull out a gold pocket watch
that dangled from a long chain
and glittered like his front tooth.
He glanced at the time
and wide eyed like a professor
quizzing his students asked,
"Boys, when's the two o'clock bus
gonna leave from Chipp'wa Falls?"
We stammered, shifted our feet
and answered, "Well..two o'clock."
"Natu'lly, natu'lly," he said,
chuckling while he walked away.

One night, at closing time,
a bartender found him,
dead in a tavern basement,
the back of his head gashed.
Some said it was an accident,
that he had fallen down the stairs,
but the gold watch he loved
so much had disappeared.
Whatever happened to Zack,
the only black man in town?

A New Man?

Local tavern owners took up a collection
and purchased a kidney for him--
what bliss! He fared so well
he once again could down a six pack
and not get up at night to piss.

When his own heart failed,
pounding wildly against his chest,
the Society of Spare Parts
donated one that lulled him
to sleep with slow and steady beats.

Corneal transplants followed,
reversing dimness brought on
by years of leering at every skirt in town--
his peepers became so keen he could spot
a set of knockers half a block away.

But after he had a stroke
and his brain was replaced,
he drank warm milk instead of booze,
paid no attention to his pulse,
ogled books instead of babes
and asked the addled strangers around him,
"Are you sure you have the right person?"

The Home

An aide draws all the shades,
an orderly dims all the lights,
someone shuffles down the hall,
somebody mumbles behind a door.

Birthday

As you always do
the day before Christmas,
you open the scrapbook
to a familiar headline
in an old newspaper clipping--
"Baby Jane Doe, a newborn,
abandoned at local hospital."
Beneath the caption, a picture of her
with tiny fingers reaching out,
her mouth a bawling circle.
You pat the face on the page
as though to quiet the infant,
as though to reassure her.
The story still overwhelms you--
snowy footprints that holiday eve,
the surprised nurse who found her
in a box inside the back door,
the note pinned to her blanket.
You linger over the details,
longing for the lost pieces
in the puzzle of a life
that began thirty years ago.
You close the scrapbook
but the same questions haunt you--
if you ever find your mother,
will she want to see you?
Who are you? Why?

My Wardrobe

I unwind a scarf of adverbs,
toss it to the side
and turn my coat inside out
in search of the proper noun.
I discard a shirt full of cliches
and empty all my pockets,
groping for the right verb.
By the time even a hint
of a metaphor rolls around
my clothes are on the floor
and I am standing in a corner
in the same old birthday suit.
When all seems lost I do
what I should have at the start--
close my eyes and try to *see,*
cover my ears and try to *hear.*

The Dying Man

The entourage that fills the room
probes and sounds the dying man
and all his divisible parts
are claimed and accounted for.

The first chants an incantation,
reaches deeply into his bag
and removes a vial of mystic cells.
He says, "It's blood he needs."

The second grasps a golden knife,
holds it high for all to see
and sweeps it through the air.
He says, "Out with his spleen."

The third peers into the inner eye,
finds a single thread and tugs,
unravelling a clew of dreams.
He says, "Dementia, don't you see?"

When they depart,
the dying man lifts his heart,
holds each chamber to his ear
and wrapped in a white sheet,
rises and begins to dance.

The Marrow's Memory

I have seen the X-rays
of those children's bones--
cracked and bowed extremities,
zigzag skull fractures,
displaced growth plates,
the broken clavicles and ribs.

I have seen the shrouds
of calcium being laid down,
the new bone that wraps
around the sites of injury
as skeletons mend themselves.
After many weeks, the evidence
of trauma usually disappears
and the bones seem whole again.

But I can not see
in any shadows before me
the marrow's memory,
the soul within the bones
that never forgets
the fist and boot,
the kicks and blows.

Leading Lady

The couple exited the cafe,
the woman, straight and tall,
with a crown of silver hair.
Her gloved hand at his elbow,
along the avenue they came
beneath a basilica of trees.
She nodded as they passed--
the distance between us grew
and I heard the city claim
the rhythmic click of heels,
the fading shuffle of shoes.

Career Choices

My friends have asked
if I went into medicine
because of the prestige,
was it to help mankind,

did research interest me?
These were considerations
but I have a confession to make--
the real reason was Roger Borovoy.

In the sixth grade after class,
we had a fist fight--my first and last.
While I peppered him with jabs
and showed off my fancy footwork,

a vision of the middleweight champ,
Tony Zale, flashed before me
and I was certain that
the boys pressed in around us

were witnessing an epic bout.
Roger Borovoy, short and squat,
pawed the floor with a heavy boot
and waited for an opening--

like Jake Lamotta, the raging bull,
he lowered his head and charged,

knocked me on my ass
and pummelled me with lefts and rights.

Had my brother not yanked him off,
my noggin would still be bouncing
on the floor of the Normal School.
I trudged home with a puffy lip,

a case of damaged pride,
and told my skeptical father
I had run into a couple of boards,
neglecting to mention

they were inside a pair of fists.
Why did I become a doctor?
Whenever someone asks,
I smile and rub my lower lip,
aware of how I would have fared
in another line of work.

Fond Remembrance

I was walking down a corridor
in the clinic where I work
when the pair of elderly ladies
in front of me stopped.
One peered at a photograph
in a row of pictures on the wall
and as she studied the bald pate
and wrinkled visage of a deceased doctor,
I imagined she was remembering
a miraculous cure of long ago,
perhaps an all night vigil
at the bedside of her relative
when house calls were commonplace,
maybe years of faithful service
he had provided the community.
Pointing a bony finger at the frame,
she turned to her friend,
thumped a cane on the floor
and announced, "That's the one
that just about did Vernon in."

Mediterranean Sunset

Born in Italy by the sea,
the spinster who taught for years
on a barren North Dakota plain
possessed the manner and look
of a schoolmarm, I thought--
so formal and dispassionate,
her brunette hair pulled back,
a pair of delicate bifocals
perched on a narrow nose.
The final time I visited her,
while searching for words
that might allay her pain,
the end of a conversation
drifted into the hospital room--
two women reminiscing in the hall
about their former beaus.
One confessed, "I don't know
what I ever saw in him.
He was a waste of time."
When their busy voices fades away,
the lady from Anzio said,
"I never spoke that way
about the men I knew.
I loved them all,
everyone of them."
Her face blossomed as if
a wild and solitary rose

had suddenly bloomed
within a fallow field.
Finally, I could see
what had always been before me--
she set her glasses aside,
reached up, untied her hair
and let it tumble
to her bared shoulders.

Rescued

I was an intern
called to the pediatric ward
to see a two year old
in respiratory distress,
teetering on her elbows and knees,
wheezing and cyanotic.
The nurse had readied a tray
in the event of a tracheotomy,
a procedure I had never performed
in an adult, let alone a child.
Suddenly, the girl toppled forward
and stopped breathing.
The nurse handed me a scalpel,
ran to the phone and had the operator
page the surgical resident on call--
"Dr. Wilson, Dr. Wilson,
Stat, Room 121, Stat, Room 121!"
I stood motionless,
terrible moments ticking away,
the knife shiny and surreal,
clutched in a hand that seemed
to belong to someone else.
Dr. Wilson charged in,
grabbed the scalpel
and jumped onto the bed,
straddling the girl as he cut
an opening in the trachea

and slipped a tube inside.
"Breathe! Breathe!" he yelled,
compressing and releasing her chest
as if it were a small accordion.
At last, a gasp--
a tide of air
swished through the tube
and she began to breathe again,
those rhythmic sounds a haunting melody
I've heard a hundred times since then.

The Summer Solstice

You showed me the mammogram
and pointed to a white star
in the dark sky of my breast--
how innocent and far away it seemed,
a sparkle on the horizon,
but I could tell that you, stargazer,
had seen that heavenly sign many times.
When you excised the cancer,
no bigger than a fingertip,
I saw the red glare of my incision,
a half moon reflected in your glasses.
No need to remove my breast, you said--
had you done so how could I have filled
the emptiness, the darkness of space?
Heal my wound the way Heracles
had his charioteer, Iolaus,
seal the gashes of Hydra.
I need your magic,
not your strength.

The Widow Speaks

Doctor, thank you
for taking care of my husband.
We trusted you and understood
whatever could be done was done.
You did explain the chemotherapy,
detailed the possible side effects,
discussed survival rates--
so professional, so complete.
I'm sure that everything
you said was true
but isn't there a way that you
can tell a man he's dying
and still leave him with hope?

Beneath a Golden Arch

The signs were unmistakable--
the acquaintance, long a steady soul,
raided his pension fund to buy
a flaming red Corvette,
began to flaunt gold chains,
auditioned for a hair transplant,
praying the tufts around his ears
would impress the dermatologist.
Instead of pizza and beer for lunch
he ordered veggie snacks,
enlisted in the Y brigade
and wheezed around the block,
attempting to deflate a pair of spares.
As for his wife, who raised their kids
and helped pay off his college bills,
he said, "No spark there anymore"--
leaving us to wonder who needed flint.
Divorce pending, he cavorted
with a pony tailed secretary
who graduated in his daughter's class.
But something happened on the way
to Cabo San Lucas and Mazatlan--
he maxed out his credit cards,
his senorita dumped him for Jose,
a guitarist in a mariachi band,
and when he called home collect,
his wife suggested he stay in Tijuana.

He did return and when I saw him last
he was dining alone beneath a golden arch
on two Big Macs and a sack of fries,
his banged up Chevy in the parking lot.

From the Earth Itself

Sunrise.
Why am I standing here,
in this valley where
a generation ago I saw
so many of you fall and where
your blood was washed away,
your faces white as snow?

I could not find you
in public places, in the stones
and monuments, and still I dream
of bones piled high and ask myself
why our swords were forged
so proudly on our fathers' anvils.

And by tomorrow, what will come
of all the promises made today?
Who will stoke the fires
and who will shape the blades?
At last, here where the trumpets blew,
I hear you in the wind that stirs,
the litany of your whispered names
arising from the earth itself.

A Fiftieth Anniversary Interview
-for the Navy flight nurses

Where shall I begin?

I was a small town girl
who had never been out of Wisconsin
until I graduated from high school.
The farthest I had travelled
was to a basketball tournament in Madison
as a cheerleader my senior year.
When the bus rolled into the capital
I was amazed at the number of people.

Medicine always interested me--
my uncle was a country doctor
who practiced forty years in Sawyer County.
I will never forget the first time
he let me look into his black bag
when I was a child. How fascinating--
listening to my heart
after he placed a stethoscope on my chest
and when he checked his own blood pressure
I watched the needle rise, then fall.
How I giggled when he made my knee
jump with a small reflex hammer.
I would have loved to become a doctor
but remember in those days
what was expected of women.

When I finished nursing school,
the thought of going overseas to care
for our troops sounded so romantic.
My father told me not to enlist--
he said it was too dangerous
but a twenty-one year old girl
doesn't worry about what might go wrong.
He gave me the gold chain and cross
that belonged to my grandmother--
you see, I'm still wearing it.

For flight nurses training
the Navy sent us to Alameda, California,
and afterwards flew us to Hawaii
and from there we went to Guam
where they had set up a tent hospital.
We made several flights to Iwo Jima,
a place I had never heard of until
we received our final orders.
The corpsman showed where it was
on the map of the western Pacific.
When we flew in on my first trip,
I looked over the pilot's shoulder
and as the island came into view
he pointed to Mt. Suribachi--
it reminded me of a great pyramid
that was rising out of a blue desert.
Could anyone have guessed how famous
that mountain would become?

We landed on a small air strip,
surrounded by casualties,
but could only jam two dozen litters
of the injured into the C47.
All we had to treat the marines
were Sulfa and Morphine,
units of blood, bandages and dressings--
and a plane full of prayers.
The corpsman and I worked together--
I wouldn't have made it without him.
We did our best for them
but how could anyone have been
prepared for what we saw?

Young men, some of them boys, really,
with head wounds, shrapnel injuries
to the chest and abdomen,
burns that blistered and oozed,
limbs that were shredded.
I knew some of the extremities
could not be saved but always told
the wounded we had the best surgeons
in the world waiting for them--
at times it's better to keep
part of the truth within you.

On one flight in March of 1945
two of the air-lifted men died

but I left their faces uncovered
and went on talking to them
like I did all the others,
not wanting anyone to give up.
The survivors didn't discover
what had happened until we arrived
in Guam and unloaded the plane.
They held my hand then,
hugged me and thanked me.

I had the same dream
over and over again--
the war had ended and we nurses
were riding a night train home.
The radio was playing my favorite song,
Doris Day singing, "Sentimental Journey."
But then her voice trailed away
and when I looked out the window and saw
the way the lights were flashing by
I realized the train was speeding backward.
"Where are we going?"
I yelled to the conductor.
"Back to where you came from,"
he answered and I began to cry.

I don't know why the tears
flowed only in my dreams--
I had held them back for so long

while we were stationed in Guam
that part of me withered
and not until returning to the States
was I able to cry again.

Whenever I see the photograph
of the marines hoisting our flag
on Iwo Jima I think of the corpsman,
the roar of the engines,
the precious cargo.

This is what I remember--
yes, put it in your newspaper.
Tell our story.

Dolly's Woes

"The DNA in her cells shows telltale signs of wear."
                                    The Associated Press

Nobody bothered me until last year.
I munched away in the fields,
not worrying about a thing,
feeling pretty because the guys
were giving me the look.
But then Doc Jitter, our vet,
started poking me for blood
and whispering to his pals.
Three months ago, over the hill,
before I could even say baaa
I was surrounded by a herd,
reporters clicking cameras,
and right behind then a bunch
of professor types ran around
like they were nuts and yelled,
"Dolly, you're a clone!"
They put my picture in the paper
and said that I might live forever
but no one bothered to ask
if that was OK with me.
At first I liked the attention
but changed my mind real quick.
The gals are jealous now
and none will chew the cud with me.

I got no privacy, can't even pee
without some jerk standing guard.
My Rambo found another squeeze--
he couldn't stand the fuss
whenever he came to see me
and says I ain't frisky anymore.
This sheep is feeling old.

The Houses That He Entered

The man who swore by Apollo
and all the other gods
and goddesses that bear witness
has at last laid down his staff.

Often in his dreams a serpent,
once cleaved by a sword,
slides across a flowered adytum
to rest a leaf upon his brow.

On awakening he sees
the paleness of his hands
instead of Glaucus stolen
from the darkest kingdom.

He closes the doors
to the temple of Asclepios,
drawing strength not from its splendor
but from all the houses that he entered.

The Ailing Poem

The poem was overwhelmed
by all my trusted therapies,
weighted down with attention
and unnecessary medication,
never allowed to free itself
of its restraints, to rise
on its own from the sickbed,
perhaps to even levitate.

And in the end,
or was it the beginning,
I could not bring myself
to bury the ailing poem.
I salvaged a phrase or two,
set flame to what remained
and fanned the fire
with all my breath.

Other Candle Lights (2008)

Grippe

A winter evening, 1916.
Anna and her husband, Niko,
with their two month old, Eleni,
bundled in her mother's lap,

rode on the train to Chicago
in search of the *mammi,*
the midwife they were told
might save the baby's life.

When they arrived
and hurried through the depot throng,
Niko handed a cab driver a note
and pointed to the address

their Priest had jotted down.
He nodded and drove them
to an old apartment where they found
the woman they were searching for,

middle aged and razor thin,
with penetrating, hazel colored eyes.
In their native language, Greek,
Anna described Eleni's malady--

a fever five days old,
a cough which had grown worse,

and lethargy so severe she couldn't suckle
at her mother's breast.

The *mammi* led them to the kitchenette,
washed her forearms and hands,
draped a clean sheet over the tabletop,
had Anna lay the infant down.

She felt the baby's brow,
noted her parched skin and florid face,
the bluish hue around her lips,
bent low and listened to the congestion,

like the sound of water
bubbling through a tube.
The midwife crossed herself,
shook her head and said,

"Grippe,"
the word as cold and hard as stone.
She told her fellow immigrants
there was nothing she could do

and in a voice subdued
added a final sentence--
"The pethani to koritsi sou"--
"Your girl is going to die."

Soon after the crowded train

hissed out of the station,
Eleni, cradled in her mother's arms,
went limp and sighed,

a wisp of wind that faded in the night
and marked the passing of her storm.
When Anna began to weep,
Niko leaned toward her and whispered,

"Don't cry now--
pretend she's still alive.
We don't want anyone to think
we didn't take good care of her."

Consumed

Before departing for America,
a young seaman, Antoni,
vowed to return and marry Irini,
a beautiful seventeen year old.

Two months after her lover left,
she realized she was pregnant
and sent him frantic letters,
none of which he answered.

She conjured up her father's face
and shuddered at the thought
of the blaze that would have raged in him
if he were still alive.

When her condition showed,
Irini confined herself to the house
and languished weeks on end,
listening to her mother wail,

"O Antonis se halase!
Ti tha kanoume?
Antoni ruined you!
What are we to do!

Once the arduous labor began,
Irini muffled her screams with a towel.

Her mother, a former midwife,
delivered a stillborn boy that night.

In the morning a fisherman
found him floating near the pier,
the umbilical cord around his neck.
No one claimed the remains.

At the baby's funeral,
O Papathaskalos, the teacher-priest,
railed before the iconostasis
that the sinners would answer to God.

Two years later, Antoni died,
consumed by tuberculosis.
His relatives took up a collection
and sent his body back to Greece

where it was interred
in the shadow of the island church
beside a small, unmarked grave.
Irini never married.

Letting Go

The rod's poised--
a snap of my wrist propels the lure
which rides in a tunnel of air
and touches down,
minnow-like and motionless,
afloat beside a lily pad.

I gather up the line's slack,
wait several moments,
twitch the lure--
the surface swirls--
a largemouth leaps and shakes its head,
trying to dislodge the hooks.

I reel the bass up to the boat,
grasp the lower jaw
between my index finger and thumb,
extract the metal barbs and hold it high,

a five pounder flaring the dorsal fin,
belly gold and gills aflame,
stark against the shoreline green
of pine and spruce and linden leaves.

I lower the fish into the lake,
letting go,
watch the bass

fan its tail and glide away,
blending with the water's hue.

So Near, So Far Away

For five years, beginning in '33,
unless inclement weather kept them home,
the father and son drove fifty miles
along a county road lined with pines

to see the boy's mother at the sanitarium
where forty TB patients were confined,
a sprawling citadel two stories high
that overlooked the countryside.

Not allowed within her room,
the youngster played outdoors
until his father's visit ended,
then ran to her window sill

and raised the pictures he had drawn
for her the week before in school.
His mother held him in her gaze,
a blood tinged hanky out of sight.

They learned to read each other's lips.
She praised his artistry
and when the time to part arrived,
they laid their fingers on the pane,
as though their hands were joined.

The Times

-for Bess

Forgive me
for the times
I did not listen to
what you had to say,
for the times
I did not listen to what
you had to say,
for the times
I did not listen to what you
had to say.

Rejoice
in the times I recognized a different
accent among the syllables of your embrace,
in the times I noticed the various ways
your hands spoke to one another,
in the times I understood
the phrases in your eyes.

The Epidemic

The summer of '45.
Aunt Lola's call was like a knife--
"Come quick, my Danny's sick,
the doctor says it's bulbar polio."
Aunt Katie and Yiayia,
who had been visiting us,
boarded the next train
with Mother for Beloit.
Not waiting there
for a connecting bus,
they hitchhiked twenty miles
in a Good Samaritan's car
to my grandparent's house
and hurried up the flight of stairs.
When they heard Papouli
trudging toward the door,
they knew they were too late.
"Ehasame to paithi," he whispered,
as if the words were blades--
"We lost the boy."

The Islander's Autopsy

—after Elytis

Renowned for its intensity,
Ionian light, the blue and white
enisled within his eye,
illuminates the retina.

A tuft of chamomile
is anchored on his tongue
and scents of basil and oregano
arise from deep within the lungs.

A maroon hue
suffuses his fingertips,
the blush which they absorbed
caressing breasts in many ports.

In the seashell of his inner ear,
one can hear a bouzouki's lament,
the clicking beat of castanets
and the rustle of a beaded skirt.

Cerebrospinal fluid
that bathes his brain
contains traces of plankton
which have washed ashore.

A garland of anemones
encircles the pericardium
and from an ancient olive tree
a thorn's imbedded in his heart.

Deep Vein Thrombosis

Harry Agganis,
the young Red Sox first baseman,
had been sidelined with a cough,
shortness of breath and chest pain,
an illness team physicians
attributed to pneumonia.

On June 27, 1955,
six weeks after symptoms had begun,
attendants lifted him into a chair
beside his hospital bed--

a clot, dark and serpentine,
dislodged from a deep leg vein,
slithered in a stream of blood
and encroached upon his heart,
obstructed the pulmonary artery
and killed the "Golden Greek."

What We Need to Know

1968,
Pediatric Clinic,
U.S. Naval Hospital,
Camp Pendleton, California.

A frazzled mother of four,
her three year old in tow,
expressed concern about her son
to Dr. Jackson, the pediatrician.

Her youngest often shed his clothes
and sped outside to play,
pausing long enough to toss
his plastic toys onto the roof.

"He's always on the go--
I can't keep up with him.
You think that he might be--
well, a hyperactive child?"

The doctor reached out,
lifted the boy and set him on his lap.
While examining the tot,
he asked her several questions--

yes, she said, he sleeps soundly,
is quiet when she reads to him

and interacts well with his siblings,
no, he doesn't rush through meals.

"From your description,
you certainly have an active child,
but hyperactive, no," the doctor said.
"He's been sitting here with me

for several minutes now,
which tells us what we need to know.
No medication or tests are necessary.
Your boy will be just fine."
How right he was.

A Narrow Beam of Light

Her father, a widower,
sits in a local nursing home,
tethered to a chair and when
his daughter tries to feed him,
he calls her by her mother's name.

"Dad, it's me, Penelope,
open up your mouth,"
she implores, raising a spoon
to form an O with her lips,
"This is good for you,"--
as soon as they escape,
the words reverberate—

his curved back straightened
and trembling fingers still,
her father stands before her,
pointing at her plate.
When she shakes her head
he flexes his biceps and asks,

"You know how I got this?"
After a dramatic pause,
he announces, "Vegetables!"
They laugh as little hands
engird the muscle in his sleeve.

Now, when she repeats the word,
a narrow beam of light
streams into her father's night
and he looks up at her as if
she had returned from a long journey.

Reaching out,
he touches her upper arm.
Before she can remind him
of all the places they have been,
his moon and stars begin to fail
and once again they are a galaxy apart.

Different Directions

At Fiftieth and Security,
while I was jingling all my coins,
she wheeled around the corner store
and glided by on roller blades
in a tank top and shorts,
a lass with long and lissome legs,
her hair a windblown flame
and breasts an orchard's best.
I would have traded in CD's
and tossed my checkbook to the gods,
if I could have turned around
and rendezvoused with her
at Seventeenth and Sunrise.

All About Harry

*"Some friend will write in the small notices
that poor Ouranis died abroad untimely."*
Kostas Ouranis

Haralambos, or Harry as we called him,
returned to Athens in a wooden box,
a forty year old neurosurgeon
who had vowed to countless women
that he would marry one of them.
With the physique of a middle guard,
intelligent and likable but coarse
and prone to eruptions during stress,
he smoked his cigarettes to the nub
and sated himself on mounds of pastries,
resolving during caloric lulls
to pare a few kilos from his beefy frame.
Aware of having heart disease,
according to local legend he refused
a coronary bypass, contending that
the heart he had would have to do.
Soccer football, as he called it,
was his favorite sport--
who could forget the Greek
with the mustache and ebon hair
lumbering down the field
as though it were his private turf.
One night while playing racquetball

he toppled to the floor
like a hewn Corinthian oak.
At his funeral, a blond nurse
came sobbing down the aisle,
consoled by another woman
who was a paradigm of serenity.
I later asked if the one distraught
was the nurse engaged to Harry.
"No" a confidant replied,
"she was his girl friend,
the other was his fiancee."

Parkinson's Disease

A swarm of pigeons flutter down
as soon as he enters the park.
Easing onto a bench,
he empties a bag of crumbs.
While birds bob and peck at his feet,
he sits, expressionless and still,
except for a hand in his lap
trembling to its own rhythms.

In the school yard across the street
the children run and skip and jump.
When the noon hour ends
and they return to class,
he lifts himself, one stage at a time,
unfolding like a wooden chair.
Tilted forward, arms tight to his side,
he starts for home, a shoe untied
as he shambles down the shady walk.

What a Life I've Had

George, a senior citizen
and son of a Lebanese peddler,
owned a successful carpet store.
He toiled in a Greek's shoe shine shop
in Sioux Falls, South Dakota
as a young teen in the 1920's
and also delivered newspapers
before he went to school,
fetching them at 2AM
when the local train arrived.

The evening of the senior prom,
he posed for a photograph--
a youth with a pile of curly hair,
a big smile on his swarthy face
and holding hands with a petite blond.
To celebrate the event,
his uncle let him use his Ford
but when George tried to start the car,
the crank recoiled and shattered his arm,
a bony shard protruding through the skin.
A doctor had to cut away the sleeve
in order to removed the sports coat.

Sixty years later, George told me,
"Can you believe it, Doc?
Three years on the job

and never had a day off
but I give credit to the Greek--
he taught me how to work.
I saved two thousand dollars
before I had the accident,
a lot of money then.
It went to pay the doctor bills
for three operations on my arm
but I never let it get me down.
"What a life I've had," he said,
chuckling as he pointed to the scar
extending from his elbow to his wrist.

Why a Grandma Pappas Saw the Priest

Gentlemen, call now
and you'll receive Rejuvenate.
The number, 1-800-Sky-High--
request our special rate!

You'll stand out in any crowd
and find yourself on top once more.
One pill will boost your self esteem,
your confidence will soar.

Rejuvenate is bound to satisfy,
so give yourself the lift you need
and even if you're over seventy,
four hour erections guaranteed!

The Fare

The taxi driver strode past
the sign that read For Sale
and when he rang the bell,
an older woman, wan and thin,
emerged with suitcase in hand,
a bandana wound around her head.
"I've several stops," she said.
"Take your time, I'll sit in back."

At 7th Street and O,
she pointed to a small brick house.
"That's where we used to live.
Although our neighborhood was poor,
this was a happy place, full of energy,
made up of mostly immigrants,
hard workers up and down the block.
My parents came from Greece in 1912
and it took five years for them
to save enough for a down payment.
They raised five children here."

In front of Central High, she said,
"How strange that as I've aged,
the memories of this school
have surfaced more and more--
classmates, teachers, sports events.
I've often thought of Jim O'Shea,

a player on our football team
who never knew how much I cared for him.
He joined the Marines and not until
our fortieth reunion did we meet again--
a widower, still handsome, I might add.
While we were dancing, he confessed
he'd wanted to take me to the prom
but didn't ask because he thought
I would have turned him down.
My father wouldn't have let me go--
my two sisters and I were not allowed
to date in high school but oh,
I wish that Jim had called."

Studying her in the mirror,
the cabbie turned the meter off and said,
"I married a gal I knew since second grade--
nothing worked the way we thought it would.
Lucky that there were no kids.
We got divorced and here I am,
a bachelor at fifty-two.

Last week I saw a lady at the mall
who lived across the street
until her husband died.
She's my age and came right up
and smiled and we talked for quite a while.
I'm thinking about calling her.
We both could use some company

but I don't want to get hurt again."

"Get on the phone, it's not too late.
Remember Frank Sinatra's song
about the second time around?
I had my chances, never married,
always looking for the perfect man.
My father wanted to arrange
a wedding with a Greek boy--
I never did agree to that."

At a deserted factory,
a shell with boarded windows and doors,
the walls emblazoned with graffiti,
she said, "Up on the second floor,
I sewed labels on shirts and coats,
received twelve dollars a week,
happy to be paid that much,
a job that helped to buy my books
when I enrolled at Normal School.
Like many older Greeks,
my parents thought there was no need
for girls to go to college
but when I earned my teacher's degree,
they both were very proud of me--
neither went beyond fourth grade.
My father liked to tell his friends,
I was an 'educated woman.'"

The driver knew the final stop,
over the bridge, across the river,
the hospice where his aunt had died.
"How much do I owe you?"
"This one's on me," he replied
and walked her to the door.
He set her suitcase down and asked,
"Is it OK to come and visit you? "
"I'd like that very much," she said
 and put her arms around him.

Unaware

"The last one's here.
A nurse put down a tube--
the poor man's out of it,"
the technician cautioned me.
The patient, grizzled and stuporous
on the X-ray table, stared at the wall.
Explaining what I had to do,
I told myself he didn't understand
and concentrated on the monitor.
As barium flowed through the tube,
I studied the stomach's curvature,
the gastric folds and shades of grey,
the filling and slow emptying,
all within the normal range.
Near the end of the exam,
I said, out of habit, "I'm almost done."
He turned his head, lifted a hand,
motioned for me to come close.
When I bent over him, he offered up
a whisper, "So am I."

Atrial Fibrillation

During the echocardiogram,
my heart's cadence sounded like
a hobbled horse clopping
down a cobblestone street.

Y Scenes

To my right, Marlon Barbella,
his muscles bulging in a tank top
two sizes too small, yells,
"No pain, no gain," at his partner, Stella,
sagging under a carload of weights.

At center stage, leering at himself
in a row of mirrors, Pecs Peerlus,
who looks away from the glass on the hour
to ward off the dreaded optic strain
that's known as hypnomesmerosis.

And on the left, beside the doll
with the ear plugs is Grunten Grohn,
a Berliner who makes us all aware
of when he presses fifteen pounds
or more above his head.

Polly Darton, jogging toward me
with a new pair of headlights
that would look good on any Olds,
has just returned from a seminar--
"California Dreaming"
sponsored by her plastic surgeon--
why did she wait this long?

Joe Sensubel, my pal
who's pedalling next to me as if
he's wearing concrete shoes,
wheezes, "Johnny, ain't this fun?
One beer or two when we are done?"
I catch my breath and say,
"Joe, the first one's on me."

In the Third Person

Jim, a retired Navy officer,
afflicted with a progressive form
of spinocerebellar ataxia,
braced himself on a walker
as he lurched to the dinner table.

His spouse, Maria,
minced the meat on his plate.
He swallowed with difficulty
and slurred the few words he spoke.
She didn't fuss over her husband
and while conversing with my wife and me,
referred to him in the third person,
as if the man she'd married wasn't there.

The next morning at breakfast,
as soon as Jim
plopped onto a chair,
a sentence, understandable,
tumbled out of him--
"I dreamt I could talk."

Consider, If You Will (2010)

That Hubbard Girl

I am the daughter not mentioned in the poem.
My father left our cold and angry home
when I was small, leaving me with Mother
and that demanding dog that I would rather
forget--she gave him wine, a hat, a fish,
fulfilled his every peculiar whim and wish,
but if I asked for even a biscuit, she'd shout
that I would have to learn to do without.

I've tried my best to not lay all the blame
on her but a story like ours should never be.
She's been dead for years and still I see
that dog lying in her lap, while I sat
praying for a hug, at least a pat,
waiting for a bone that never came.

Bluebeard's Therapist

Youthful psychic traumas, we now know,
may recur in adults, to their dismay.
Your mother's disappearance long ago
may be heightening your sense of loss today.
I'm sure that you will find another wife--
who knows where the prior ones have gone.
Don't agitate yourself, get on with life,
it's best to deal with loss and move along.

As for those quiet spells you've set aside,
continue on with them, relaxing hours
behind closed palace doors where you reside.
Next time, tell me more about that room of yours,
the one with trophies hanging on the wall,
where you enjoy your pipe most of all.

A Shadow of Himself

What a spectacle, a sad charade,
the naked emperor who was on parade.
A ruler, once so visionary and bold,
came to believe whatever he was told
and revelled in imaginary clothes.
Why were we so blind, do you suppose?
Was it only the power of suggestion,
were we afraid to ask a simple question?

It took a child to break the spell and see
him as he truly is, a parody,
a shadow of himself. Without delay,
return him to the castle, that we may
remember him the way he was, as though
he's still the emperor of long ago.

The Injection

Doc, by now I bet you must have heard
the name I'm called--"loser" is the word.
Who wants to be remembered for second place?
I'll never figure out that stupid race.
Whenever I come across that lowdown reptile,
he winks and then gives me a phony smile
and says, "Another chance? I'm all heart.
I'll even let you have a bigger head start."

I know that none of this makes any sense.
The rematch is tomorrow, no use pretending
I'm not afraid I'll lose again to the tortoise--
I'd rather have a case of rigor mortis.
This story's got to have a different ending.
Doc, I need a shot of confidence.

The Long Winter

The giant built the wall to keep them out,
the children who were running all about,
trampling grass and stepping on his flowers
while playing in his garden countless hours.
No longer would he share the apple trees
and hummingbirds, the butterflies and bees.
Where is his spring this year? No tulips now,
no lilies seen, no leaves upon a bough.

Beyond the wall, the robins carol long,
the fields and hillsides bloom, as if in song,
but in his garden where there's little light,
the earth is bare, no melodies delight.
Although he's come to loathe the stone divide,
his massive hands are helpless at his side.

The Little Match Girl

Were you among the throng that lined the street
and passed the youngster huddled by the door
without a coat, no shoes to warm her feet?
Every precious match she struck, she swore
would be the last but soon most all had burned.
Not a single sale--what would she do,
suffering her father's wrath if she returned
with empty hands and not a cent or two.

The tiny flares evoked a Christmas scene
upon the wall, a rush of gold and green.
Then high above, she saw a shooting star--
was it a sign, a calling from afar?
She lit the final one, a burst of light--
who took her in their arms that wintry night?

The Disappearance

Your Lucy Gray's been gone for years and yet
the coachman swears that when the sun has set
she dances in the mist that shrouds the fen,
a shepherd hears her singing in the glen.
An angler claims he's seen a little girl
with ashen face and locks of amber curl
along the river darting past the willow
where her footprints ended in the snow.

And you, her parents, what do you believe?
How long must one endure the dagger's thrust,
a wound so deep that you will always grieve?
And if one day a buckle turned to rust
is found, a shoe or bone now bleached and bare,
would that disclosure lessen your despair?

The Cure

Peter forced his wife for years to bake
him pumpkin pies and pumpkin bread each day
without a word of praise, for heaven's sake.
One March fifteenth, when she began to bay,
the priest performed an exorcism, no less,
a gypsy brought her cards to fortune tell,
and leeches were applied, without success,
so Peter put her in a pumpkin shell

and sold her to a canine circus show.
The howling ceased that evening, wouldn't you know.
When the promoter claimed a breech of contract,
she told him Peter was the one to contact.
Within a week, the ex-pumpkineer ran off
with the German shepherd trainer, Gunther Hoff.

Performances

Revered by all and known as Old King Cole,
his servants tend to each of his requests.
They scurry for his slippers, pipe, and bowl,
decant the vineyard's best for all his guests.
The jesters entertain the royal gatherings
the way their fathers did so long ago,
the jugglers toss their wooden pins and rings
and minstrels sing the tunes he used to know.

Inheriting a crown but not the temperament
to reign, the aging king of merriment
who yearned to live a life his very own
now nods and dodders on an ancient throne.
No longer able to laugh, he smiles upon
his subjects as the fiddlers three play on.

Possessed

Shipwrecked, I was washed ashore,
where Calypso cared for me and what's more
she fell in love and would not let me go.
I've yearned for Ithaka but even so
could not resist an ardor so intense,
and returned her affection, without pretense.
The gods decreed she had to set me free,
and after seven years, drifting out to sea

on the raft I made, I wave farewell to her,
knowing I'll never forget such beauty and allure.
At my journey's end, will I find
the inviting wife I chose to leave behind,
when I put my arms around Penelope,
will Calypso be the one enchanting me?

In This Infernal Place

I push the stone upward, laboring,
head down, elbows locked, imploring
every sinew that I have to not relent,
but near the top I always falter, spent,
and once again it rolls back down the slope.
Then I begin anew, flushed with hope,
undaunted by the challenge of this task.
Why do I continue, you might ask.

Without the stone, how would I ever face
the endless hours in this infernal place?
Without the heavy burden and this steep hill,
how could I test the limits of my will?
I don't complain and never stop to rest.
Some day I fear that I will reach the crest.

Suppression

Circe said the sirens would be there
in wait and warned me of their song's allure.
I told my men to lash me to the mast
and plug their ears, lest all be cast
onto the jagged rocks and killed that day.
Rebuffed, the sirens plunged into the sea
and when they drowned, I thought that I was free.

How very wrong I was, for still they tax
me so, echoes in the chambers of my sleep,
and rouse in me a craving dark and deep.
Why did I need to listen to them sing?
Had I known the woes that they would bring,
I also would have filled my ears with wax.

The Ascent of Icarus

My father, Daedalus, with good intentions,
preoccupied himself with his inventions--
the lever, wedge, and maze so paramount
that I believed I was of no account.
Before we lifted off the Cretan shore,
he cautioned me and, as he had before,
predicted our escape would represent
his most ingenious accomplishment.

But it was I who rose into that glare,
higher than even he would ever dare,
a moment which for once was mine to claim,
the feat forever coupled with my name.
And even as the feathers, one by one,
wafted down, I did not curse the sun.

A Psychiatric Opinion

Why do you need to sit atop the wall,
ignoring all the dangers that are involved?
There are some other patients, I recall,
who've lived on the edge and never have resolved
their inner conflicts. This non-conformity
is a compulsive trait, a form of obsession,
perhaps a rebellion against authority--
as a child, were you forced to go to confession?

If you should tumble down from such a height,
consider the spectacle, a gruesome sight--
who would want to gather up the pieces?
Not even the King with all of his resources
could help you then. I recommend hypnosis,
a cure for many forms of psychoneurosis.

The Quiet Ones

Yes, there was a flock of us, it's true,
squished together in that smelly shoe.
The old woman always ate the bread,
while we, her children, got the broth instead,
and even though we never said a peep,
she caned us all before we went to sleep.
Now that we are grown and she has passed,
we tell ourselves those days are in the past.

We meet just once a year, at the cemetery,
up on the hill outside of Canterbury.
Sitting far apart, we picnic there,
enjoy the view, inhale the open air,
and just for fun, throw rocks at her headstone.
Then, in single file, we start for home.

Erato Returns

I wondered if you had deserted me--
you said I lack originality,
that my prosaic style did not inspire you.
I feared you had discovered someone new.
Forget the money spent on rose bouquets
I never handed out, those drawn-out days.
The evenings waiting up were even worse,
a pen in hand but not a line of verse.

Now that you are back, I must confess
it's hard to concentrate--the flimsy dress,
your cleavage on display, those fingertips
caressing every string, the ruby lips.
I'm going to give you up, but not tonight--
come lie next to me and make things right.

In the Third Season (2012)

I

Will it be an alter ego *I*,
resplendent on the trapeze,
a proxy for the look alike
who gazes from the wings?

Will it be the ventriloquist *I*,
trying not to move his lips,
content to let the marionette
entertain the crowd?

Will it be the dramatic *I*,
within the spotlight beam,
reciting a monologue in a voice
that could belong to no one else?

Will it be the unmasked *I*,
alone on the high wire,
inching forward, arms outstretched,
performing without a net?

The Music of Their Lives

The hostess, Venetia,
a lady in her eighties,
led her aged husband to his chair,
laid a napkin on his lap,
encouraged George to eat
but did not linger over him.

He nibbled at his food,
seemed not to notice us,
the other five enjoying lamb,
Greek salad and potatoes,
dished up with generous helpings
of lively conversation.

Midway through the meal,
as if he'd heard the lyrics of a song
he used to know by heart,
George looked up, gazed at his wife,
raised his glass of wine and said,
"Si yia, Venetia--"
"To your health, Venetia."

Echoing his toast, she smiled
and for a few, fleeting moments
he recognized the melody as well,
the music of their lives.

A Winner

During a coffee break,
I and several other doctors discussed
the pros and cons of chiropractors.
I recounted my mother's story

of when I was three months old
and developed severe pneumonia.
After our family physician
told my parents I might die,

they summoned the Greek Orthodox priest
from Fond du Lac to Eau Claire
where he baptized my twin, George, and me
and older brother Dale as well.

The next day, the local chiropractor,
said to possess curative powers,
came to our house, placed me prone
across his lap, drummed on my chest,

and then, my mother said,
 "A large amount of phlegm came out."
Jim Coffey, a pathologist
listening to this saga,

looking as if he had just been dealt
four aces in a high stakes poker game,

leaned toward me and asked,
"Out of you or the chiropractor?"

A Supplication

Katerina knelt beside her son,
an epileptic eight year old,
restraining him as he grew taut
and suffered through another seizure.

When the spell ended and he lay
in the unconscious state,
she sponged him with a warm cloth,
went outdoors, turned her palms upward

and beseeched the Virgin Mary,
"*Panayia,* cast this sickness out
of my boy and give it to an animal!"
Their border collie, the family pet,

edged up to her, convulsed and died.
Her son never had another episode.
To venerate the *Panayia,*
she purchased an icon of her

for the chapel on the isle of Proti,
a few kilometers from Marathos,
the Greek seashore village
where Katerina was born.

Testament

--for Dimitra, 1930-2009

When the leukemia,
smoldering for years,
flared into a raging fire,
this lady with the glowing smile
and gentle ways told me,

"I want to make it through the holidays,
so my loved ones can enjoy Christmas."
She willed herself into January
and died at home with family at her side.
Her heart survived the blaze.

Transition

He listened to his footsteps,
receding echoes in the corridor,
and when he paused, the hush
unsettled him as nothing had before.

His intellect advised, "Walk on,
the time is right to leave,"
but oh, his soul refrained,
appealing for a day's reprieve.

Estate Sale

When Martha's husband died,
a college student bought her car,
a ten year old Mercury with a mere
50,000 miles on the odometer.

As the young man began to back
the car out of her driveway,
the widow raised her arms
and yelled, "Wait a minute!"

She used her apron to wipe away
a spot of dirt on the windshield,
shook her finger and said,
"Take care of it, you hear,
my husband saved six years
so he could buy this car."

After the new owner left,
Martha's son tried to comfort her--
"Mom, we did what was best--
it was just sitting in the garage.
I'll take you anywhere you want to go."

He hugged his mother,
strolled towards his SUV
and when he turned to wave goodbye,
she pressed a hanky over her mouth

and hurried into the house.

After the Painting by Velazquez

Don Sebastian, one of many dwarfs
in the Spanish court of Philip IV,
is seated on the floor, a crimson smock
draped over his shoulders and back,
fists pressed against his belt and thighs.
Those dark, uncompromising eyes
convey an aura of intelligence--
is there also anger and impatience?

Why this composition, why this pose?
When the session ended and he rose,
returning to his jester's role once more,
was he as entertaining as before?
How many in the crowd identified
the little man the painter personified?

What's in a Name

In the bagel shop
I'd frequented for years,
I queried the new owner,
a taciturn woman from China,

"What is your name?"
"My name Susan," she replied.
"What your name?"
"John, my name is John."

She studied me, as if she were
deciphering a complicated map,
shook her head and concluded,
"You no look like John."

"Who do I look like?"
I asked with trepidation.
"You combination man,"
Susan said with certainty.

Redder Than Any Rose

-for Louis Reyes

In a St. Paul neighborhood pub,
the man they dubbed the "Gentle Giant"
buys two dozen roses from a vendor,
presents a red flower to each lady,
the way one bestows a modest gift
upon the women of royalty.
The patrons raise their drinks
and after several toasts,
he ventures out onto the city streets,
buoyed by smiles he left behind.

Three teenagers stop him.
The fourteen year old boy
wielding a shotgun demands money--
a scuffle ensues and a girl commands,
"Shoot him! Shoot him!"
He raises the barrel,
a delicate finger squeezes the trigger--
the "Gentle Giant" pitches back
and crashes on the walk.
A pool, redder than any rose,
wells around what remains
of the Viet Nam veteran.

Waiting Room

"We interrupt this show
to bring a special update,"
the commentator pants.
"According to reliable sources,
O.J. Simpson, the movie star
and football legend, is a suspect
in the brutal murders of his wife
and her male companion."

The waiting room crowd stirs
and everyone stares at the TV,
except a mother and her girl,
a teen slumped in a wheelchair,
blue eyes askew, head lolling like a doll's.

The mother strokes the daughter's hair
and pats her withered arms.
A door swings open and the nurse
emerges with a heavy chart and says,
"Susan's next, Mrs. Person."

As the mother lifts herself from a chair,
the man seated next to them
tugs at his Dodger's cap,
leans toward his wife and divines,
"No way O.J.'s guilty--he's my hero.
You can't find them anymore."

At the Organ Bank

I'm back
and strapped for cash,
just like before.

What do you mean,
no kidneys needed now?
That's all I have to give.

See this glass eye--
I should have got
at least another grand.

Wouldn't have sold my leg
if I knew how clumsy
a wooden one would be.

Remember the Cherokee
I paid for with a lung?
It's been repossessed.

For Christ's sake,
I sold my colon
to pay my son's tuition

and traded in my spleen
so we could go to Spain.
I'm all used up!

What? Are you for real?
Not that, no way,
not in a million years!
What'd you say
the guy would pay?
A Rockefeller, for sure.

Let me use your phone--
if the Mrs. says OK
we got a deal.

Wishes

A tubing winds down
from a bottle of glucose
to join a catheter that snakes
into a vein in a woman's hand.
A man beside the bed
withdraws a potion from a vial,
injects it into the solution
and opens wide the clamp--
the drip becomes a stream.

A voice booms over the intercom,
"Code blue, room 222! Code blue, room 222!"--
in seconds the CPR team
thunders past the door.
When the bottle is half empty,
she inhales through pursed lips,
as if trying to cling to a bubble
shrinking at the end of a straw.
She gasps the last word,
"Wait!"

He waits five minutes, uncoils
a stethoscope and listens to her chest
as the final hint of color fades
from his patient's face.
He glances at his watch,
signs the proper document

and dials the nurse.
"Dr. Sleighton in 201.
Please notify the son--
he's waiting for the call."

Secret Formula

-- *Nation's oldest person dies at 113.*
                              Associated Press.

In a San Pablo nursing home,
a spinster, Mary Christian,
recalled the San Francisco earthquake
which occurred when she was 17.

A few months before she died,
a reporter, wondering how
she had reached such an advanced age,
bellowed into her ear,
trying to extract an explanation
from this antique.

Was it because she abstained
from alcohol, disdained tobacco,
refrained from vulgar language,
did a tranquil disposition
account for her longevity?

She shook her head and said,
"It was none of that--
Twinkies and Kentucky Fried Chicken
kept me going this long."

The Ultra Ultrasound

The doctor peers into a watery world,
the transducer in his hand a beam
sounding the depths for a pearl
lustrous enough for even a queen.

He samples the fluid and declares,
"No abnormal configurations allowed,
no translocations, and every pair
of chromosomes must be properly endowed."

The computer whirrs and gleans,
a breathless minute for the mother to be--
the screen lights up like a marquee--
"The Perfect Baby! The Perfect Baby!"

She blushes and confesses,
"That's what we've wanted always--
do we buy pants or dresses?"
The doctor frowns and says,

"It really doesn't matter.
You can't keep the baby--
we've been waiting much longer.
Next time, be lucky."

As Is

The middle aged mechanic,
riddled with metastases,
sat in the doctor's office
as the oncologist discussed the need
for yet another cancer drug
in hopes of stemming the disease.

Hands quiet in his lap,
the stricken man stared
at blotches on his arms,
silent until he rose to leave.
"Doc, do you know anyone
who wants to buy an '80 Ford?"

The Siamese Twins

When he awoke and found
that Chang had died during the night,
did Eng succumb within the hour
because of shock and fright?

Was the loss of vital force
an anatomic certainty, the event
peculiar to their conjoint state,
a reversal one could not prevent?

Or had there been a wish fulfilled,
a tacit covenant between the two,
the bond that tethered them
a crossing death could not undo?

To Sound His Name

Although he still performed
with aptitude and zest,
the elder surgeon opted to retire
because his hearing loss progressed.

He feared an error might occur--
a word not registered
or number out of range,
a cautionary voice not heard.

He dreams of the operating room,
returning to a familiar well
to sound his name and plumb the depth,
to end another arid spell.

Person to Person

Professional white male
with movie star features,
middle aged but look much younger,
great conversationalist and dancer,
pro-feminist, ISO of single woman,
age 30-65, less than 5'6",
financially independent.
Race and looks unimportant.
A golden opportunity
that others missed--
don't let it happen to you!
Include photograph. Box 10.

Dear Mr. 10:
Saw your ad in the <u>Minnesota Trapper.</u>
Am self employed, a full figured widow
considered attractive by some.
Enjoy reading, walks, the lakes
but you sound like the munchkin
psychologist with elevator shoes
I had a blind date with last year,
the one who stepped on my toes
at the St. Mary's singles dance,
talked for hours and borrowed cab fare.
Send *your* picture first. Box 100.

With Steadied Hands

When the auto crashed,
the young man was dashed
against the steering wheel.
Chest X-rays suggested
a tear of the aortic wall.

As we prepared for the angiogram,
his parents arrived and found him
lying on a cart in our radiology room.
The father, overcome, turned away
as the mother leaned over their son
and squeezed his hand--
"We're here, Jim, we're here..."
His eyes fluttered open--
"Mom and Dad, I'm not ready to die!"

His declaration filled a cup
we shared with steadied hands.

Peripatetic

He speeds along ignoring all
the flashing lights and warning signs--
arterial avenues clog with plaque,
cerebral intersections atrophy,
people's names veer off Memory Road,
boulevards of bone collapse.
His favorite interstate has exit ramps
that only lead to dead end streets.

Sages say that age is but a state of mind
but when the peripatetic shaves
he can not help but see unfold,
in a creased and weathered map,
a California of yesterdays,
a Rhode Island of tomorrows.

Found Poem at Board Meetings

HMO
need for different logo

corporate culture
how to be a team player

capitation
reducing over-utilization

improving efficiency
performance of collection agency

eliminating discounts
preferred accounts

raising co-payments
encouraging retirements

increasing market share
strengths of managed care

recruiting new physicians
profit sharing and pensions

new business manager
employee vs. employer

doctors' parking lot design
the bottom line

outpatients

Instruction

An English class for refugees--
I sat in back, a volunteer
who watched the teacher try
to elicit the word, "tree,"
from the disparate group,

among them Somalians, Sudanese,
Bosnians and Vietnamese.
She shaped a circle in the air,
fluttering fingers meant
to represent a crown of leaves.

Not yet obtaining a response,
she chalked an image on the board,
a globe shaped like a cauliflower
perched atop a slender trunk.
Again, she queried them,

"What is this a picture of?"
A young man from Srebrenica,
tapping his feet beside me,
answered in a voice so subdued
I was the only one who heard the word,
"Bomb."

He Set Aside the Instruments

Because of a retinal mass,
suspicious for malignancy,
a specialist referred my wife
to a renowned ophthalmologist,

grey haired and tall, near seventy,
his demeanor deferential and calm.
For quarter of an hour he gazed
through a phoropter into her eye.

Employing a hand held lens,
he then defined the lesion's depth,
diameter, its margin's clarity,
the nature of the pigmentation.

Proceeding with his evaluation,
he gently pressed a transducer
against the sclera, by ultrasound
defining further the abnormality.

His examination complete,
he set aside the instruments,
folded his arms and stood before my wife.
"This is benign," he said,
"A nevus, not a melanoma,"
his words as welcome as the air.

Mistaken Identity

After reviewing a scan
with a comely gastroenterologist,
a new addition to our clinic,
I asked how her family had adjusted
to their recent move.

She replied, "We've done fine
and I am very fortunate.
If I had to live my life over again,
I'd do everything the same."

She studied the photograph
on my desk of my wife and me
and our four children who then
were in their teens and early twenties,
both daughters seated by my wife,
our two sons standing behind them,
yours truly perched on the sofa's arm.

"A fine picture," she noted.
"I see you have five children."
Pointing to my spouse, I sputtered,
"But...but... that one's my wife."
Unabashed, she said,
"How nice, how very nice."

Just Like a Tree

Until the giant came to town
that day in May of 1940
when I was ten years old,
nothing exciting happened
in our town, Bulan, Kentucky.

Dad said, "Wear your Sunday dress--
were going to see Robert Wadlow,
8 feet 11 inches, the tallest man
who ever walked the earth."

A huge crowd was waiting in front
of Smiths Store, where they sold
the brand of shoes the giant wore.
Someone took a picture of us kids
while we were on the balcony next door
and put it in the newspaper--
I was the one in white.

When their car pulled up,
the giant's father was the driver.
They'd taken out part of the front seat
so the giant could sit in back
with room to stretch his legs.

It seemed to take forever
for him to get out of the car

and as he did, I saw his shoes,
size 37, the window poster said.
When he straightened up,
you could hear the oohs and ahs.
I was surprised he used a cane
and walked real slow, like an old man.
Wouldn't you know,
right away someone asked,
"How's the air up there?"

Dad was standing close to him,
looking up and shaking his head
like he couldn't believe his eyes.
The store owner came outside
and greeted the giant like a king.

After staying for an hour,
he squeezed back into the car,
took off his hat and wiped his glasses,
a blond haired, tired looking man.
As they drove away, Dad said,
"I've never seen such a thing."
That's all he talked about for weeks.

A few months later,
after coming home from work,
Dad said he wasn't hungry.
When Mom asked him what was wrong,
he showed us the newspaper article—

the giant, who was only twenty-two,
had died of blood poisoning
while he was on tour in Michigan.
His leg brace had rubbed against his foot
and caused a blister that got infected.

Robert Wadlow was buried
in his hometown of Alton, Illinois.
Forty thousand people came to his funeral.
Dad kept saying, "I don't believe it--
he was a miracle, just like a tree."

The Cancer Patient

I know
the feel of monitors,
drains and catheters,
tubes of every kind,
bandages that bind.

I do not know
if anyone has time
to lay their hands on mine.

Untitled Poem

In the midst of errands, preoccupied,
I strode along the downtown walk,
unmindful of the June cerulean sky,
the zephyr wafting through the trees,
the choreography of leafy shadows.

A young man limped toward me,
his right side partially paralyzed,
a surgical scar above one ear.
As he labored by, he said,
"Beautiful day, isn't it?"

So Long

When Kenji was twenty-five,
Japanese officials sentenced him
to spend the remainder of his life
at a Nagashima Island leprosarium.

Stigmata of the disease
marked him in the ensuing years--
scattered nodules, loss of fingertips,
a nasal deformity and lopsided face.

In 1988, the government built
a bridge across the narrow waterway
which separates the island
from Honshu on the mainland.

Kenji, seventy by then, vowed
to see the other side before he died.
A public education campaign
encouraged local citizenry

to welcome island lepers,
none contagious, all on medication.
Stooped and white haired,
dragging a duffel bag of clothes,

he trudged across the bridge,

a span of only fifty yards.
Arriving at the cleaner's store,
he set his laundry on the countertop.

The owner, her back toward him,
turned and when she saw his face,
covered her mouth with a cloth,
grabbed a pair of wooden tongs,

shoved the bundle back at him
and pointed toward the door.
As he retraced his steps,
Nagashima's iron bell began to knell,

invoking memories of home
for those who have been gone so long.
Kenji pinned a note to his bag,
left it at the leprosarium

and trudged upward toward the peak
above the Inland Sea to face the west
from whence the lepers came,
the route to heaven, Buddhists say.

Facade

Before my heart began
skipping beats and racing along,
an aura of invincibility
had wrapped me in its armor.

These paroxysms grew
more insistent and prolonged,
arrhythmic bursts
pounding on my metal chest

until each rivet popped,
the springs and hinges sprung
and a facade of iron plates
fell clanging at my feet.

The Sinister Hand

Between Barstow and Las Vegas,
eastward bound for home
some sixteen hundred miles away,
I was humming a radio tune
on a cloudless April day at noon
as the car was zooming down
the interstate on cruise control.

My left hand, resting on my knee,
suddenly tingled, as if electrified--
I looked down and saw
two left hands,
one a phantom image,
the other reaching for me

seemed alien, disconnected,
an intruder's hand--
"No!" I yelled--
a moment later images fused
and only then did I recognize
my hand, my hand!

Illusions

In cardiac intensive care
after my coronary bypass surgery,
I saw two imps on tricycles
pedalling in the room,

a regiment of white ants,
in single file, inched across
the ceiling toward a combat zone,
each one's pincers armed
with a grain of sand,

this while an unseen hand
set in motion the framed print
that dangled on the wall
beside the bed I occupied.

On the third post-op day,
the tots and trikes disappeared,
the ant brigade returned
to its barracks underground
and the picture ceased to move.
I was sound again.

Scarlet Fever

--Mother's story

In 1926, when I was eight,
Mama and Papa couldn't afford
two cents to buy us milk at school.
A friend shared hers one day

and sure enough, we both got sick.
The Health Department came
and tacked a sign on the door,
a two month quarantine.

My throat was red and very sore,
and I was so feverish
Mama had to sponge me down.
A rash spread all over me

and a week went by
before it started to fade.
I'll never forget the way the skin
peeled off my feet.

While I was sick, Papa gave me a doll
with reddish hair and skinny legs.
She looked like Raggedy Ann
and I was proud of her.

I called down to the kids outside,
lowered her from the third floor window
on a string I tied around her waist.
Papa said that they could look

but weren't supposed to touch.
There she was in front of them--
you should have seen their faces then,
the open mouths and eyes so big.

That was seventy years ago
but seems like yesterday.
I don't know what happened to my doll,
the only one I ever had.

Achilles

Now that our wooden horse has led the way
and we have breached the Trojan walls and gate.
I remember the prophecy I'd die on the day
an arrow, guided by Apollo, sealed my fate.
Surely, this can not be the gods' intent,
so l will celebrate this time and place.
Our well earned victory is imminent--
let the vanquished live with their disgrace.

When I was an infant, my mother dipped me
in the waters of the River Styx.
Since then I've been invulnerable, a mix
of fire and steel, fearful of no enemy.
Look at Paris drawing back his bow--
how meaningless, a gesture meant for show.

Rightful Owner

Months after the transplant,
the recipient quit the medication
prescribed for him, required
in order to prevent rejection.

The hand that once belonged
to someone else became
more swollen and grotesque,
the hue of a blue-red flame.

When he insisted that
the surgeon remove the hand,
the doctor appealed to him,
"Don't you understand,

this was the first of its kind.
I've explained the reasons why
we have to follow protocol.
Think of the time my team and I

have spent preparing for this--
I will not undo my surgery."
The patient raised the hand and asked,
"Does it belong to you or me?"

Sunny Days

An older woman in a dark blue dress,
her white cane leading the way,
edged up to me after my poetry reading
at the Braille Institute yesterday

and reminisced about the time
when she had won first prize
in a high school English class
for her poem, "Summer Skies."

As she recited the opening line,
light came shining through the haze
and the radiance of old returned,
her eyes as bright as sunny days.

Circle Dance

Bea, ninety-seven years young,
beamed as she reminisced
about her father, once a minister
in Mt. Carmel, Illinois.

"He liked to call me his pal,
a five or six year old who tagged along
when he went downtown to visit friends.
He'd have me show them what I'd learned,

so I would raise my arms above my head,
turn slowly and begin to sing,
'I am a little prairie flower,
growing wilder by the hour...' "

Bea set her walker aside,
joined hands with that little girl
and they whirled in a field
which glowed with goldenrods.

His Good Stuff (2017)

Last at Bat

He checked each box score
as a boy, baseball games
the day and night before.

Now, in his 79th year,
on reading the local tabloid,
scans obituaries for a familiar

name, perhaps an old colleague
who collapsed while rounding first
in the Senior Citizens League,

or a geezer who went down
while he was limping out
a dribbler past the mound.

Maybe Slivers passed away,
the guy who rode our bench,
praying for a chance to play,

or perhaps the shortstop, Matt,
took one for the team,
a fast ball in his last at bat.

Just in Case

At the Metrodome in the late 80s,
a small crowd showed up for the game
between the Yankees and Twins,
a pair of also rans that year.

Wheelchairs were commonplace
and an entrance sign read that
the handicapped would be honored
on that weekday afternoon.

I sat in the stands between home plate
and first base and to my left a fivesome
was sporting Iowa T shirts and caps—
two adult men, two boys in their early teens,

probably their sons, and an older man
who could pass as the grandfather,
missing two fingers of his right hand.
Before the game began seven men,

including two with Down's Syndrome,
sat directly in front of me,
flanked by a male and female attendant.
A few innings into the contest,

the batter hit a foul pop up
which bounced in the nearby isle

and caromed toward the Iowans—
a lad of theirs leaped up,

caught the ball and held it high
to show the fans nearby.
A man in the disabled group
extended his palm and said, "ball,"

but when the lucky boy
handed it to him to look at,
he turned and hurled the souvenir
back onto the playing field.

"Oh, no!" the male attendant yelled,
and as if prepared for such contingencies,
reached into his jacket and removed
a shiny baseball which was passed along

and given to the crestfallen son
who had just lost his memento.
One of the Hawkeye fathers rose,
approached the guilty party,

zeroed in with his camera, took one,
and then another picture of the man,
bent forward, elbows on his lap,
hands covering his face.

Power Outage

A switch hitter, Rocky, relied on a pack
of syringes delivered in a small paper sack—
when he exhausted this glandular array
no matter how hard he would swing away
his balls petered out on the warning track.

Refreshments

—Veeck's Midget Plan Was Picture Perfect.
                              Chicago Tribune

The irrepressible owner
of the St. Louis Browns,
Bill Veeck, who lost a leg in WWII,
loved capers and clowns.

He conjured up ways to lure fans
to games of his team, dwellers
oftentimes in the dimmest corners
of American League cellars.

On August 19, 1951,
before the second baseball
game of a doubleheader with Detroit,
a 26 year old man, 3'7" tall

and wearing a batboy's uniform,
popped out of a large plastic cake
in front of the Browns dugout
and proceeded to make

his way to the on deck circle,
The announcer said, "No. 1/8,

Eddie Gaedel, batting for Saucier."
When he came to home plate

pinch hitting for the leadoff man,
the ump refused to let him bat
but when the Browns manager
produced a contract that

had been signed by Veeck,
he allowed Gaedel to step into
the batter's box. The owner had told
him he was not to

swing at any offering of Bob Cain,
the Tiger hurler, who lobbed four straight
high pitches to his catcher, Bob Swift,
on his knees behind the plate.

Gaedel headed for first base
after he received the free pass
and bowed to the delighted crowd.
"I felt like Babe Ruth," he told the press.

When he reached the bag, a pinch runner,
primed and prepped for the occasion,
replaced Gaedel who left the field
and received a standing ovation.

A few days later, Will Harridge,
President of the American League,
voided the contract and ruled that midgets
could not play in the big leagues.

Gaedel earned $100 for his appearance
and $17,000 for promotions and interviews,
including Veeck hiring him as a vendor,
"who wouldn't block the fans' views."

He died in 1961, his name
etched in the record book stats,
one of five players who reached base
in their only major league at bats.

His pinch hitting appearance
highlighted one of the worst
seasons the Browns ever had.
They finished 46 games out of first.

Next time you're at the ball park,
look for a little guy in the aisles
beside an older fella with a wooden leg,
working the stands, wearing big smiles,

hustling candy, $10 beer, and peanuts,
call out as soon as they're in range,

be sure you buy two of everything
and tell them to keep the change.

Her Moment of Bliss

On June 14, 1949,
while the Phillies played the Cubs
at Wrigley Field on Ladies Day,
Ruth Steinhagen, nineteen,
sat spellbound in the stands,
rekindling a blaze that she possessed,

fixing Eddie Waitkus in her gaze,
the handsome first baseman
Chicago had traded to Philadelphia
before the season had begun.
She'd pored over sports pages,
sliced his pictures out of magazines,
the man she had never met,
a World War II combat vet,
recipient of four Bronze stars.

That night she reserved a room
at the Edgewater Beach Hotel,
knowing he'd be there,
imploring him to meet with her--
she had a message, she said,
one that couldn't wait.

Shortly before midnight,
a knocking at the door--
ushering him into the room,
the tall brunette excused herself
and fetched a rifle from the closet.
"Is this some kind of joke?" he asked.
She pulled the trigger--

a bullet ripped into his chest
and as he slumped to the floor
had strength enough to ask,
"Baby, what'd you do that for?"
She notified the operator
who summoned the hotel doctor
and in her moment of bliss,
the one she'd craved so long,
Steinhagen held her idol's hand.

At the Cook County jail,
she relished the barrage
of questions reporters fired at her,
their pens and pencils poised.
Informed Waitkus had survived,
she said, "I dream of him every night,"
and pointing to his pictures in the cell
asked, "Why is he always smiling?"

174

Room for Improvement

"It usually manifests itself as an inability
to throw the baseball accurately"

I knew a catcher from St. Kitts,
who developed a case of the yips,
so severe that he could not throw
the ball to any base and so
he studied other cases for tips

on how to cope with this vexation—
the Sax and Knoblauch situation,
the trials of Steve Blass and Jon Lester.
He underwent hypnosis, acupuncture,
and a neuro-psychiatric evaluation,

all for naught but a San Jose
trainer cured him in a single day
when he advised , "Forget one size fits all,
what you been wearing's way too small—
go buy yourself a bigger cup, today!

Ode to a Closer

Dan Quisenberry, 45, died yesterday.
N.Y. Times, October 1, 1998.

The Kansas City Royals bullpen ace
appeared in two World Series in the 80's,
not overpowering, but he possessed
the best control in the Major Leagues
and showcased a submarine delivery,
his money pitches sinkers that coaxed
a host of ground ball outs.

Players, fans and writers admired
this right hander with the red mustache,
a modest man who credited team mates
when he snuffed out rallies and shunned
excuses if he failed to save a game.

A quipster and wordsmith
with a wry sense of humor,
he served up memorable quotes—
"I found a delivery in my flaw,"
"I want to thank the pitchers
who couldn't go nine innings,"
 and describing his Peggy Lee fastball said,

"Is that all there is?"

Toward the end of his pitching career,
he furthered an interest in poetry,
enrolled in writers' workshops
where he shared his verse,
surprising many followers
who had never guessed
he nurtured a creative bent.

In 1998, shortly after learning that
he had a cancer of the brain,
his book, On Days Like This,
was published, free style verse,
direct and economical, as in
the tribute to his former manager—
Dick said he was tired
go on without him
baseball's just a game
try to win...

In the late innings of his malignancy,
after trials of surgery and chemotherapy,
he was asked if he wondered, "Why me?"
Dan Quisenberry said, "Why not me,"

as though he had just retired the side
and was walking off the mound
with the game ball in hand
and a poem in his back pocket.

Side by Side

The southpaw, Tommy John,
tantalized batters with slow balls
he kept low while carving corners
of the plate with sliders and sinkers,

inducing grounders and double plays,
frustrating hitters, in particular
free swingers who tried to drive
his pitches out of the park.

While with the L.A. Dodgers in 1974,
he tore the medial collateral ligament
of his left elbow, which usually meant
the end of a hurler's playing days.

An orthopedic surgeon, Frank Jobe,
suggested he best give up the game
but this athlete wanted to compete again.
The doctor offered to perform

a procedure not done before--
he would transplant a tendon
from the pitcher's right wrist
to his injured elbow and drill holes

in two bones to secure the graft,
hoping it would stabilize the joint
and function like a healthy ligament.
He informed Tommy John

the chances he'd be able to pitch
afterwards were "one in a hundred"
but his patient insisted they proceed
and underwent the experiment.

The lefty spent a year in recovery,
adhered to a careful rehab program
and rested his arm for months
before picking up a ball again.

In 1976, Tommy John returned,
toed the rubber on the mound
and showed players and fans
he could still get batters out.

This battler from Terra Haute
went on to win 164 more games,
a total of 288 big league wins
in a span of 26 years.

He retired from the sport in 1989.
On July 27, 2113, in a ceremony
at the Baseball Hall of Fame
in Cooperstown, New York,

as they stood side by side,
Tommy John introduced Frank Jobe,
the unassuming North Carolinian
and decorated WW II veteran,
honored for pioneering the surgery
which resurrected many careers.

Bottom of the Ninth

When he was young,
the slugger seldom walked
and won many important games
by belting long home runs.

An oldster now
with cancer in his liver and lungs,
he checks out the scoreboard,
steps into the batters box
and takes three called strikes.

His Most Important Saves

In the late 50's, Ryne Duren,
the big Yankee relief pitcher
with 100 mile an hour fast balls
was often summoned by the manager,
Casey Stengel, to close out games.

He would vault over the bullpen fence
along the right field line,
amble to the mound, peer down at the plate
through thick dark glasses and uncork
a warm up pitch onto the backstop screen,

reinforcing his reputation as
a reliever with poor control
and even poorer eyesight
who dared batters to dig in
when they stepped up to bat.

He had a short but effective career
with the Bronx Bombers,
a four time All Star who appeared
in the World Series as well.
More important than his baseball stats,

when his playing days came to a close,
he learned to tame the throes

of depression and drinking sprees
which had plagued him
most of his baseball career.

He lent his name to support groups,
made many public appearances
and counseled other alcoholics.
Years after Ryne Duren left the game,
he made his most important saves.

Undeterred

Jim Abbott, the big southpaw
born without a right hand,
starred at the U. of Michigan
and 1988 Olympic games.
He played in the big leagues ten years
and in his finest season won 18 games
for the California Angels.

He learned through trial and error
to rest the glove on his right forearm
and after he released the pitch
would slide his hand into the mitt,
ready to field his position.

After catching a batted ball,
he trapped the mitt between his chest
and right arm and in one motion
slipped his hand out of the glove
and removed the ball,
ready to throw to any base.

In New York on September 4, 1993,
while pitching for the Yankees
against the Cleveland Indians,
Abbott hurled a no hitter and when
the final batter grounded out

his teammates raced to the mound and mobbed him as 27,000 fans cheered for the man who pitched as if he had two hands.

One Pitch Away

August 16, 1920,
a grey, overcast day
at New York's Polo Grounds.
The Yankee, Carl Mays,

a righty with good control
who relied on a submarine delivery,
which when combined with dirt and spit
on the ball made it hard for hitters to see

the pitch as it left the hurler's hand.
Cleveland Indian shortstop, Ray Chapman,
a right hander who stood close to the plate,
was batting in the fifth inning when

Mays threw a pitch that struck him
in the left temple, the sound
a thud so loud that when the ball
rebounded toward the mound

Mays thought it had caromed off
Chapman's bat and threw the ball
to first but when he turned
and saw the batter sag, then fall

to his knees, blood streaming out
of his left ear, he realized

he had hit Chapman in the head.
Carried off the field and hospitalized,

his condition worsened
and doctors performed surgery
which revealed a fractured temporal bone
and a blood clot due to a torn artery.

He died the following day,
the only Major League fatality
which occurred as the result
of an on the field injury.

Mays insisted he had thrown a strike
and said the fact that Chapman
hadn't leaned away from the plate meant
he didn't see the pitch zooming toward him.

Several witnesses agreed
but some Cleveland players wanted Mays
out of baseball—their manager did not agree.
Mays was exonerated by the Manhattan's DA.

The Indians regrouped and went on
to win the pennant and World Series that year.
They voted to give Chapman's pregnant wife
 her husband's winning share.

His death ended the dead ball era.
Spit balls were outlawed with some exceptions
and when dirt or scuffs appeared on baseballs,
they were exchanged for new ones.

Carl Mays won 207 games during his career
but fell short of the votes required for induction
into the Hall of Fame. After his playing days,
he spent twenty years as a baseball scout
and died in California in 1971, one pitch away
from being remembered as a very good pitcher.

Lou Gehrig's Disease

*Amyotrophic lateral sclerosis (ALS) is
a motor neuron disease that effects
voluntary muscles, causing atrophy,
weakness and paralysis.*

On May 2, 1939, in Detroit,
before the Yankees played the Tigers,
Lou Gehrig walked slowly toward
home plate and handed the umpires
New York's starting lineup.

They were amazed to discover
his name was not included on
the card, the first time that occurred
since he became their star first baseman
in 1925, a span of 2130 games.

He had spoken with Joe McCarthy,
the team manager, earlier that day
and told him he would remove himself
from the lineup because of his poor play
which had begun the previous year—

a loss of power at the plate,
inability to drive runners in,
unsteadiness on the base paths,
difficulty fielding his position
and impaired reflexes.

A few months later, on July 4,
he gave his farewell speech to the fans
at Yankee Stadium and said in part,
"I consider myself to be the luckiest man
on the face of this earth..."
The Iron Horse had come up lame
and never played another game.

That Changes You

Lou Brissie, an All Star, dies at 89.
New York Times, Nov. 26, 2013

In the summer of 1940
a tall seventeen year old lefty
from South Carolina who possessed
a sharp curve and a big fastball
drew the attention of baseball scouts
and the Philadelphia Athletics manager,
Connie Mack, who advised him
to finish college and then try out
for his American League team.

The war intervened and he joined
the Army's 8th infantry division,
stationed in northern Italy
where it experienced heavy casualties.
German artillery bombarded his unit
on December 7, 1944, killing eleven soldiers,
and when a shell exploded near his feet,
shrapnel shattered Brissie's shin bone,
the left tibia, a jigsaw of fractures, the wound
laid open and infection prone.

When taken to a Naples hospital,
surgeons noted the contamination

of the injury site and recommended that
the young corporal undergo an amputation—
"Don't take my leg off, I'm a ball player," he said
and they agreed to try to save his limb.

Brissie endured two dozen operations,
refused medication for constant pain,
walked with crutches for many months
and then began to throw a baseball again,
lobs at first, regaining balance and strength,
wearing a heavy metal brace to support
his leg, two inches shorter than the right.

In 1947, after two years of rehab,
he won 23 minor league games
and Connie Mack called him up
to the Athletics at the end of the season.
In the next two summers he notched
30 victories and fulfilled a lifelong dream
in 1949 by pitching three innings for
the American League All star team,
alongside players whom he idolized,
like the shortstop, Lou Boudreau,
and two fair to midland outfielders,
Ted Williams and Joe DiMaggio.

He retired from the game in 1953,
became one of the coordinators

of American Legion junior baseball,
helped establish sports programs
in Australia and Latin America.

A baseball scout for several years,
he later worked for the state board
of South Carolina, training workers
who had applied for new jobs.

Brissie required follow up care
at VA hospitals the rest of his life,
often seen several times a year,
on crutches, the leg painful and deformed.
A doctor once approached him
about making a movie to chronicle his life.
He nixed the idea, saying,"I left a lot of guys
in the hospital—it wouldn't feel right."

A reticent man, he found a way
to encourage veterans who had sustained
a myriad of injuries in Iraq and Afghanistan.
Interviewed many times, Brissie said,
"Things that look impossible are not.
People with disabilities have told me
I inspired them—that changes you."

The On Deck Circle

Dorothy Kamenshek, who helped inspire
the lead character in "A League of Their Own,"
has died. AP Press, May 23, 2010

When my brother and I
visited our relatives in the 1940s,
aunts and uncles took us out to see
the Rockford Peaches, one of the teams in the
All American Girls Professional Baseball League
that operated from 1943 to 1954.

Sixty-five years later, in 2007
in Palm Desert, California, we met
for the first time their star first baseman,
Dorothy Kamenshek, an 84 year old
in a wheelchair who joined us for lunch.
Her teammates called her Kammie,
to distinguish her from several players
who were also named Dorothy.

Soft spoken, steady handed and alert,
she reminisced about the times
her widowed mother, on the way to work,
would drop her off at a Cincinnati park
where boys enjoyed playing baseball.
At first averse to the southpaw joining in,
they changed their minds when they saw

how well she played the game.

Invited to a Wrigley Field tryout
in 1943 at the age of seventeen,
she made the final cut and joined
the Rockford squad, the anchor team
in the league that included cities like
Grand Rapids, Kenosha, Racine,
Kalamazoo and Fort Wayne.

An All Star several times, she won
two batting titles and Wally Pipp,
the Yankee player, said that she
was the best fielding first baseman,
man or woman, he had ever seen.
Sports Illustrated in 1999 selected her
as the 100th greatest female athlete
of the twentieth century.

Kammie chuckled when she recalled
lessons in etiquette given to players,
dress codes and hairdos required,
the curfews they were supposed to keep
while boarding with host families
who provided rooms for them.

Players earned $50 to $125 a week,
received an expense allowance and saw
the Great Lakes countryside by bus.

In August, 1950, three thousand fans
honored her at Beyer Stadium
in Rockford on "Kamenshek night"
and showered her with gifts.

When her playing days ended in 1953,
she attended Marquette University,
embarked on a career in physical therapy,
went on to head that department of the
Los Angeles Crippled Children's Service,
an experience she said gratified her
as much as baseball accomplishments.

Kammie gave us each an autographed photo
of herself, taken in her Rockford uniform,
was pleased that we remembered her
and delighted in revisiting the past,
as if she had risen from her wheelchair
and trotted back to the on deck circle
with her favorite bat in hand.

My Glove

Once or twice a year,
while boys are shagging balls
in the park across the street,
I, a middle aged Ponce de Leon,
rummage through the garage,
foundering in a sea of boxes.
At last I find my glove
and ease it on as I always do,
pound the pocket with my fist
and tell myself I could play today—

but I want to remember
Joe DiMaggio the way
he raced from first to third,
his graceful outfield style
and power at the plate.
Let someone else watch
an idol hobble around the bases
in an Old Timers Game.
So I return my glove to its proper place,
to be retrieved whenever I see
a ball that's spinning toward me
from my summer days.

New Poems

Leader of the Little Band

--One of the last Munchkins dies at 93.
            AP, November 17, 2011

Karl Slover, the sole dwarf in his family,
as a boy was immersed in sand and oil
by his father who then tried to stretch
his son on a machine, to no avail.

When he was nine, his father sold him
to a European troupe, the Singer Midgets,
who formed the core of a circus group
which later came to the United States.

In *The Wizard of Oz,*
he played the 4'4" trumpeter
who led the Munchkin parade
when it announced their mayor.

He and 123 other dwarfs
each earned $50 a week
for their performances
in the 1939 film classic,

which Karl liked to remind others
was less than that paid to
the canine performer of the movie,
the Cairn terrier named Toto.

He and six other Munchkins
appeared on Hollywood's Walk of Fame
in 2007 and received a collective star
and a plaque in their name.

At ease in front of cameras,
he enjoyed interviews, signed autographs,
attended reunions and festivals,
was quick to reminisce and laugh.

According to a long time friend,
Karl Slover did not understand
the meaning of the term, "stage fright."
How does one measure such a man?

So Sedate

In the mid 1940's,
Vasili, a Greek immigrant
about to return to his homeland,
lost all his savings one night
in a New York City poker game.

He soon became confused,
heard voices, dark and shrill
and could not sleep.
A childhood friend escorted him
to a psychiatric hospital where
he was confined for many weeks.

The attending physician,
citing a "lack of progress,"
authorized a surgical castration
because of "persistent melancholia."
A few months after this procedure,
the gloom enshrouding Vasili
lifted and he regained his sanity.

Friends and relatives bought
him a ticket back to Greece
and when he returned,
his siblings all agreed
that they had never seen
their brother so sedate.

The Second Best Thing

At the Gyros Bar and Grill,
Panos, my philosopher friend,
asked me how I'd like to go
when my days are over with.

I said it's for the gods
to understand these things
but if I could choose
the way to leave this life,

number one would be
to take the last breath
in my woman's arms
just after we made love.

The second best thing,
to end up like Brando did
in *The Godfather* when he
was playing with his grandson

and fell over in the garden
between the rows of tomatoes,
back to where he came from--
the seeds, the leaves, the earth.

A Ways to Go

Overweight since childhood,
the writer tried diets, retreats,
hypnosis, exercise routines--
a repletion of defeats.

The family doctor referred her
to a specialist to see
if the patient qualified
for bypass gastric surgery.

At his office, in a gown
that didn't cover her in back,
she weighed 190 pounds.
He pointed to a chart, in black

and white and said, "You're supposed
to weigh 110—if I'm to operate,
you have to be at least 100 pounds
above this ideal body weight."

When she drove away,
an emptiness from deep inside
began to gnaw at her again,
a hunger never satisfied.

She stopped at a grocery store,
bought a pecan pie, a box of Snickers,

three cans of peanuts, a quart of ice cream.
"I have company," she told the checker.

Plodding from the car to her door,
weighted down, she could not keep
herself from thinking of Virginia Woolf,
the stones, a river cold and deep.

Flight Nurse

As they prepared for departure,
the ailing pilot glanced at the clock,
then traded places with his wife
who took over the controls
for the very first time on that,
the final stage of their voyage.

Just as the plane touched down,
the sun dipped below the skyline.
She laid her hand on his and said,
we made it home on time,
we made it home.

Like All the Rails

John Logan, ninety-three,
had worked half a century
on the Northern Pacific.
Talkative and spry, this lightweight
loved to flash his railroad card
and enjoyed reminding me,
"I go anywhere on the train, free."

Scheduled to have a cataract removed,
he asked, "Doc, what do you think
of a man my age having surgery?"
"Can you see the pretty girls?" I asked.
"You bet and I still look," he replied.

After his admission on the eve
before the tentative operation,
he became confused, tried to climb
over the railing of the hospital bed,
tumbled to the floor and broke his hip.

The injury required surgery,
a repair with screws and a metal plate.
A month later, he died at home,
his cataract in tact,
the fracture well aligned,
like all the rails John Logan laid.

Detours

As the older couple entered the cafe,
he clasped his lady's hand
and steered her to a booth.
His bright blue T shirt read,
"Walk a mile for Alzheimers."

He patted her on the arm,
proceeded to the counter
and ordered their breakfast,
his manner calm and resolute,

a man who looked as if
he had studied the map
and was prepared to navigate
the detours they'd have to take
on their way back home.

Scoliosis

A photograph,
Circa, 1925,
Erikousa, Greece.

Spero, our paternal grandfather,
and Thea Sophia, his daughter,
gaze at the camera lens,
arms linked, expressions stern,

a lean cigar in his left hand
and a tie tucked under the vest
of his baggy suit. Behind them,
in the shadows, a calico cat
explores a rocky slope.

His torso's torqued,
one shoulder droops,
signs of spinal curvature
common in men who form
our branch of the Manesis tree.

MRI

Readied for the brain scan,
I lie supine, ear plugs inserted,
the ceiling scene a quietude--
a lake, a grove of trees.

A support, a hockey mask of sorts
with openings for the eyes,
keeps my head still.
The tech slides the table into
the machine's tight circle.

I close my eyes
and silently recite three poems,
calming ones about my grandparents
and Thea Kati, the story teller,

the background noise a fan
that's droning on and on,
interrupted by sequenced staccatos--
the woodpecker on my left
bangs on a pole, then a pause,

the jackhammer answers on the right,
pounding on a metal plate
and when these competing sounds rest,
I hear a washing machine in the rinse cycle,
this sequence repeated again and again.

The tech cautions me, "a little stick,"
injects gadolinium into my arm vein.
A shorter round of sounds and I am done—
the exam "just 23 minutes," he says.

Why Now?

Our father disapproved
of my mustache and goatee
and more than once opined,
"That's not the way
a doctor's supposed to look."

In 1979, when my wife and I
were planning a trip to Greece,
including a visit to Erikousa,
the islet where he was born,

I asked what he'd like for us
to bring him when we returned.
He said, "I don't need a thing,
just do me a favor, please—
before you go, shave."

I did not heed his advice
until two years later, shortly before
I went to see him in the hospital
and sensed it was a final opportunity.

On that, our last reunion,
he was oriented and alert,
and refrained from commenting on
the change in my appearance.

I wonder if he asked himself,
why now?

KO'd

September 23, 1952,
World Heavyweight Championship,
Municipal Stadium, Philadelphia

In the 13th round,
the champ, Joe Walcott,
well ahead on points,
starts to throw a punch—

Rocky Marciano plants his left foot
and with all 188 pounds
behind his right hand cross
wallops Walcott on the jaw—
his head snaps back and to the side,

he sags face down,
onto the lower ropes,
suspended,
motionless,
unconscious,
counted out.

What He Meant

When I was a student nurse,
the instructor told our class one day,
"Hearing is the last sense to go--
be very careful what you say."

In intensive care after my fall
I couldn't move or see yet somehow
heard my doctor tell a resident,
"It's just a matter of time now—

she's been comatose a week."
I tried to call out, to be heard,
to ask him what he meant,
but could not say a word.

Deciding Vote, 1954

--for my twin brother

Our father wanted George and me
to attend the local Denver University
after high school graduation and what's more
expected us to continue working at his store

but we dreamed of going to Boulder
where girls gave guys a warm shoulder
and we could party every night,
enjoy the scenery and delight

in downing 3.2 beer with buddies
at a popular pub called Tulagi's.
When we suggested that venue to
our father, a grade school graduate who

earned a degree in practical economics,
we stressed its beneficial academics
and painted an optimistic rendition
of an out of town education.

He looked at us like a loan officer
dealing with a no-collateral customer
and made this proclamation
without further deliberation--

"Go to Boulder, you pay,
stay in Denver, I pay."

Missing Conversations

After his wife died,
a house painter in his fifties
stopped nightly at a sports bar
on the way home from work,
something he seldom did
when she was alive.

He would nurse a beer
while glancing up at ball games
on the array of TV sets,
the music in the pub so loud
he cupped an ear to hear
the friend who often joined him.

One night, the fellow worker said,
"Jim, it's way too noisy here—
let's go to Larry's Bar sometime."
The widower replied,
"We were married thirty years.
Sue liked to talk and lots of times
I nodded but didn't hear a word.
Now I hate going home—
it's so damn quiet there."

Straight Ahead

My doctor's a computer man
who says he loves the Apple store.
He looks at the monitor
and types away as fast as he can--
not much eye contact anymore.

The Only Way

When brother, George, last saw
Aunt Katie in a nursing home
near the end of her long life,
dementia had reduced her to a shell

of the vibrant lady we once knew.
Trying to jog her memory,
he reminisced about our relatives
and Rockford days when we were young.

She sat speechless, rubbing her thumb
over his black onyx ring,
a replica of one her father, our *papouli,*
had worn on special occasions,

like the time he accompanied George
to the house on Kishwaukee street
where my brother proposed
to a beautiful Greek immigrant.

Was Aunt Katie's gesture
a substitute for imprisoned words,
the only way to show that she
could touch upon the past?

Marking Her Territory

In 1971, we presented our sons
and daughters with a Christmas gift—
Tasha, a Norwegian elkhound pup,
a playful and good natured pet,

but over the course of months,
she shredded kitchen wall paper,
dug huge fox holes in our back yard
and barked and barked.

When I consulted a veterinarian
employed by the Mayo Clinic
and described our canine's tendencies,
he explained that working dogs

like ours require exercise and asked
if I had time for daily jogs with the dog.
If not, he suggested that I let her run
alongside my car on a country road.

"She's needs to vent her energy—
that's why she barks so much," he said.
I thanked him and replied,
"You told me all I need to know."

I suggested to my patient wife
the time had come to give Tasha away

but she insisted we recoup
our $35 purchase price.

A farm couple in their forties
who owned another elkhound
answered our newspaper ad.
When they entered the house,

Tasha sprinted toward the wife,
jumped up to lick her face
and peed on the lady's shoe.
"Get out the checkbook,"

she told her man and moments later,
Tasha, without a leash or backward look
bolted out the door and leaped onto
the back of their pickup truck.

I Danced to All of Them

A trim man with a grey crewcut
who looked to be in his 60's
answered my ad about the records
needed for the jukebox I had bought,
a 1947 Seeburg.

He greeted me at his door,
limped across the living room,
plopped down on the sofa
and pointed to a cardboard box
filled with 78 RPMs.

"I danced to all of them--
waltzes, rhumbas, polkas, swing,
but since my surgery,
even the two step is hard," he said,
rapping on his prosthetic leg.

I bought two dozen discs
and as I was leaving he added,
"I gave my phonograph away
but when I'm restless at night

turn the radio on beside my bed
and listen to the oldies station,
the hits from the 40's and 50's--
that's better than a sleeping pill."

High Handicaps

In my California winter golfing days,
when a new playing partner asked about
my primary residence, I confessed
to living in Fargo, North Dakota.

Invariably he would ask,
"Did you see the movie, Fargo?"
"Oh, yeah, you betcha, four times,"
I'd say then nod and look away.

If he happened to be an older vet
who had served in WWII,
another query might ensue—
"You know Joe Schmidt,

my Navy buddy in '43
from Minot, North Dakota?"
I'd shake my head and explain
that city's 270 miles west of Fargo.

He would seem disappointed,
certain the two of us must have met.
Sometimes, I heard a trailing question,
just before we got our Big Berthas out

and swung away from the red tee box
on the 150 yard par 4 first hole—

"Mount Rushmore's in North Dakota, right? I'd smile and say, "Aw, geez, you're close."

Barter, 1936

My brother and I
gave Dr. Hayes a start
when we were born
six minutes apart—

he had not expected two of us.
Our father, at his Eau Claire restaurant,
had sent Thea Kati to the hospital
with Mother and when our aunt

called and told him he was
the father of twin sons, he was sure
she must have misunderstood
what the doctor had said to her

but when he arrived at the nursery
we convinced him otherwise.
Mother's four day stay cost $200—
he suggested a compromise—

the Sisters of Sacred Heart Hospital
agreed to his proposal that he
pay off the debt with ice cream,
gallons churned by George Lemke

in the silver basement vat
of our Dor Smith Cafe,

enjoyed by patients and nuns
alike for many a day.

A 1967 California Prophet

Frisky, a Humane Society waif,
the first of a menagerie of cats
enthroned in our homes for fifty years,
fell ill soon after her she arrived,
besieged by vomiting and diarrhea,
unable to eat or drink.

An Oceanside veterinarian examined our pet,
a Marlboro dangling from his lips,
ashes littering the examining table.
Poking the feline, he drawled,
"Enteritis due to Cat Fever,
almost always fatal, ya know,
wiping out their white cells
but dehydration is what kills 'em.
Won't do this animal much good
but I'll give her a shot," he said
with a mortician's solemnity
as his needle impaled her rump.

Returning home with a hobbled pet,
I called another vet who told me how
to replace the fluid loss by clysis,
injecting saline under her skin,
which I did for several days.
To our surprise, Frisky recovered,

the lone residual a limp
related to a gimpy hind leg.

The Connection

An elder in a wheelchair
motored into Applebees
and double parked at a table
near the front door.

His right arm paralyzed,
he ordered by tapping on
a menu luncheon entry
with his left index finger.

When the food arrived
and the server set it down,
the man shook his head
and slurred, "Nuh, nuh, n--"

a second server and a manager
hurried to the scene but none
of them could understand
what he was trying to say--

one grabbed a ketchup bottle,
the second a fistful of napkins
and the third inquired,
"Potato chips instead?"

The customer jabbed the air
and pointed to the exit sign.

One of the trio guessed,
"You want this to go?"

He nodded and a minute later
wheeled out of the restaurant
with his hard earned prize,
a cheeseburger and fries.

Distance

I paused on my morning walk
when a man trimming his hedge
greeted me and went on to say,

"I enjoy working in my yard—
you see, I'm a caregiver now.
My wife's inside in a wheelchair.

We've been married fifty years.
I never leave her by herself
and when she needs to know I'm here,

she calls me on our cell phone,"
he said, patting the holder on his belt.
"Sometimes she thinks I'm miles away."

A Family Treat

—for Bea

A ninety-eight year old invited me,
my wife and our daughter to dinner
at the retirement home where
she had resided for a year.

When the server brought dessert,
dishes of vanilla ice cream,
our hostess smiled as reminisced
about those childhood days

when her father, a minister,
on occasion married couples who
had crossed the Wabash River
from Indiana to marry in Illinois—
the latter state had no waiting period.

Eight years old then,
she'd fetch a neighbor to serve as a witness,
Bea's mother would don a Sunday dress
and play a wedding song
on the old piano in the living room.

After the ceremony,
couples gave a dollar to her father
and hurried off to begin a new life.

That meant a family treat--

her father handed the money to Bea
who would run downtown
with her brother to buy
a quart of vanilla ice cream.

Nine decades later,
as she savored each spoonful
in a local dining room,
the years melted away.

To a Listener

In 1816, a French physician,
René Laennec, instead of resting his ear
on the patient's chest to evaluate
her pulmonary congestion,

listened at one end of a notebook
he rolled up and pressed against her
and discovered this maneuver
intensified the sound.

With this principle in mind,
he hollowed out a piece of wood,
ten inches long, in three sections,
and through this cedar tube

could hear the heart's refrain
and the melody of respiration
with greater clarity than ever before,
an invention which turned out to be

one of medicine's most important.
He borrowed two words from the Greek—
stethos—chest, *scopos*—discovery,
and called the instrument a stethoscope.

Properly Aged

I open up my treasure chest
this drowsy day of reverie,
pore over the collectibles
and rediscover me—

three favorite jukebox records,
Bing Crosby's *Blue Skies,*
Al Jolson's *Some Enchanted Evening,*
Vaughn Monroe's *Riders in the Sky,*

a book with poems by Dickinson,
Cavafy, Kunitz, Hay and Oliver,
short stories by Papadiamantis,
Chekhov, Flannery O'Connor,

a butterfly net and pinning board,
a spinner bait and floating lure,
the 5th Crow Wing's shoreline map,
the Kenner's gift, George's putter,

an album honoring three dogs,
one guinea pig, a host of cats
and Zip, a charred play monkey--
thank God, no rats--

our children's grade school photos,
ballet slippers, a piano exercise,

a Monopoly board and deck of cards,
two headbands from Indian Guides,

Ben Felson's radiology text,
the plaque presented to me
by our X-ray student techs,
the lead glove used in fluoroscopy,

the Littmann stethoscope
I listened with in Appleton,
the roster of Navy doctors
in '67 at Camp Pendleton,

Grant's Atlas and *Gray's Anatomy*,
my wife's engagement photograph,
the nurse's training cap she wore,
a picture of St. Joe's medical staff,

the acceptance letter I received
from Creighton Medical School,
an eight ball and ping pong paddle,
my physics class slide rule,

menus of the Normandy Cafe
and Denver's Pizza Roma,
a City Park Sundries snapshot,
my East High diploma,

a Rockford Peaches ticket stub,
copies of Latin I and II exams I took,
lightning bugs flashing in a jar,
The Twisted Claw, a Hardy Boys book,

the Eau Claire paper's snapshot
of our 6th grade softball champs,
a baseball, scuffed and worn,
an album of Greek stamps,

antique family photographs
which come to life in proper light,
our young cousin's sailor uniform,
laid to rest with him one night,

Yiayia's hand sewn tablecloth,
the missing notebook of Papouli's rhyme,
one of the drawings Mother made,
the watch that kept my father's time,

and at the bottom, from grapes
nurtured in my own vineyard,
a bottle of red wine, properly aged,
to be savored now and shared.

Notes

93. **Atrial Fibrillation.** An irregular heart rate, often rapid, sustained or intermittent, more common in older patients.

103. **The Long Winter.** A variant of Oscar Wilde's story, "The Selfish Giant."

105. **The Disappearance.** An extension of William Wordsworth's poem, "Lucy Gray."

136. **The Siamese twins.** Born in Siam in 1811, Chang and Eng settled in North Carolina where they were given the surname, Bunker. They married two sisters and sired 21 children. They died hours apart in 1874, joined by a band of tissue near the lower sternum.

146. **Just Like a Tree.** Robert Wadlow at an early age developed a pituitary benign tumor, an adenoma, which produced excessive amounts of growth hormone and was responsible for his gigantism.

151. **So Long.** In 1996, Japan repealed the law which confined leprosy patients to institutions even after they had been

cured of their disease.

154. **The Sinister Hand.** The visual disorder described is called *palinopsia,* a prolonged after image, in this case a transient mini-stroke due to a small clot formed in the heart, an embolus which travelled to the brain. The word "sinister" is derived from the Latin word meaning "left."

156. **Scarlet Fever.** This disease is caused by a Streptococcal infection, quite contagious and usually responsive to Penicillin which was not clinically available until 1941.

158. **Achilles.** The arrow found its mark and killed Achilles. When he was an infant, his mother immersed him, holding him by the heel, the only area which did not come in contact with the River Styx. Paris was the Trojan who abducted Helen.

173. **Her Moment of Bliss.** After months of rehab, Waitkus rejoined the Phillies in 1950 when they won the pennant, the beginning of the decline in his baseball career and personal life. A heavy smoker and drinker, he died of cancer in 1972. Steinhagen, diagnosed as schizophrenic,

was confined for three years in the Kankakee State Hospital, then discharged. She died in Chicago in 2013.

179. **Side by Side.** Although both John and Jobe were honored that day, neither has been selected for the Hall of Fame.

187. **One Pitch Away.** Ray Chapman was the only player in the major leagues who died of an injury incurred during a game.

190. **Lou Gehrig's Disease.** He died in 1941 of complications of ALS. His consecutive game mark was broken by Cal Ripken, Jr. of the Baltimore Orioles and stands at 2,632.

214. **KO'd.** A knockout punch, a severe cerebral concussion, causes the brain to bounce back and forth between the bony confines of the skull.

235. **To a Listener.** Laennec died of tuberculosis, the same disease that killed his mother and many of his patients.

Other Poetry Books by John Manesis

The Journey of Andrew Burke   1998

With All My Breath   2003

Other Candle Lights   2008ß

Consider, If You Will   2010

In the Third Season   2012

His Good Stuff   2017

About the Author

John Manesis, born in 1936 in Eau Claire, Wisconsin, graduated from Denver University in 1958 and Creighton Medical School in 1962. He practiced Internal Medicine for eight years, then was a Diagnostic Radiologist from 1971 until his retirement in 1996.

His poetry has appeared in over 100 literary publications, including several anthologies. He and his wife, Bess, a retired nurse, have lived in Fargo, North Dakota, since 1974. They have two daughters and two sons.